SMART
MEDICINE

SMART MEDICINE

How To Get The Most
Out Of Your Medical Checkup
And Stay Healthy

BRUCE HENSEL, M.D.

G. P. Putnam's Sons, New York

This book is designed to help you communicate more effectively with your doctor, and to provide the information necessary for you to actively participate in your own health care. This book should *not* be used to replace consultations and appropriate visits with your doctor. Responsibility for any adverse effects resulting from the use of any information contained herein is expressly disclaimed.

Throughout *Smart Medicine,* I refer to doctors as "he." This is by convention only, and is not intended to offend or imply that all doctors are male. In fact, one third of all physicians are female.

G. P. Putnam's Sons
Publishers Since 1838
200 Madison Avenue
New York, NY 10016

Illustrations copyright © by Lisa Amoroso

Library of Congress Cataloging in Publication Data

Hensel, Bruce, date.
  Smart medicine.

  Includes index.
  1. Medicine, Popular.   2. Self-care, Health.
3. Consumer education.   4. Diagnosis. I. Title.
RC81.H52   1989   613   88-32286
ISBN 0-399-13446-8

Printed in the United States of America
1   2   3   4   5   6   7   8   9   10

For my parents.
My mother, whose patience, love and devotion never wavered.
My father, whose own growth taught me the value of
introspection and honesty.

And for Jay Ira.

Acknowledgments

No book with the lofty goals of being completely valid and up-to-date while providing you with enough information to participate in your own medical care can be written without the help of friends and colleagues.

I would like to thank the following physicians for their patience, understanding, and expertise in checking the manuscripts for medical accuracy.

Michael Fischer, M.D., Associate Clinical Professor of Radiology, University of Southern California School of Medicine; Chief, Vascular and Interventional Radiology Section, Hospital of the Good Samaritan, Los Angeles.

Jeffrey Galpin, M.D., Associate Professor of Medicine, UCLA School of Medicine; Director, Porton Clinical and Medical Laboratories, Encino and Reseda, California.

David Grimes, M.D., Professor of Obstetrics, Gynecology, and Preventive Medicine, University of Southern California School of Medicine, Los Angeles.

Richard Marrs, M.D., Director, Institute of Reproductive Medicine, Hospital of the Good Samaritan, Los Angeles.

Jerrold Mink, M.D., Associate Clinical Professor of Radiology, UCLA

School of Medicine; Head, Musculo-skeletal Radiology, Cedars-Sinai Medical Center, Los Angeles.

P. K. Shah, M.D., Associate Professor of Medicine, UCLA School of Medicine; Director, In-patient Cardiology and Cardiac Care Unit, Cedars-Sinai Medical Center, Los Angeles.

Contents

Introduction

Just a few years ago, your right to know the things you will learn by reading this book—how to tell if your doctor is competent, how to determine which medical tests are appropriate for you, how to do your own physical exam—would have been challenged vehemently.

Patients were discouraged from getting too involved in their own medical care, and doctors believed that the "routine office physical" was the simplest, safest, and most cost-effective way to promote health.

But times and attitudes have changed.

The experts have discovered that your participation is far and away the most crucial factor in the prevention and cure of disease. Public training in Cardiopulmonary Resuscitation (CPR) has saved as many people from death due to sudden heart attack as all our new scientific technologies combined. Recent studies show that yearly checkups by the doctor don't always justify their expense. As a result, the American Cancer Society, the American Heart Association, and the American Medical Association now suggest that the frequency of office visits be guided by medical history and physical symptoms rather than by the calendar. For once, what makes good economic sense makes good medical sense as well.

In my fifteen years of medical practice and as a member of the media, I've found two things to be uniformly true: 1) There is no factor more important in the prevention and cure of disease than doctor-patient communication. 2) In the development of that communication, there is no factor more important than your understanding of your own body and of the medical tests and treatments that are available to you.

But scientific technology is developing at breakneck speed. With all the new options and information, you could easily reach a point where you feel overwhelmed and decide to leave the choices about examinations, medical tests, and treatments to the experts. That sort of choice could be dangerous—for your pocketbook and your health.

I receive many calls and letters from people just like you who have felt confused, frustrated, and frightened by the scientific jargon or the technical information that was supposed to improve their medical care. They've been subjected to too many risks and spent too much of their own money on inappropriate or unnecessary medical tests.

I wrote this book to help you change all that. In the process, I learned some things about myself.

In Chapter Two, I tell you a very personal story about the death of a child whom my parents had before they gave birth to me. His name was Jay Ira, and he died only two weeks after being born, probably because of the inaction of an incompetent doctor. There's no way to be sure about the circumstances—hindsight is always 20-20—but I am sure that the stories my parents told me about those times played a big role in my choosing medicine as a career. Just as I'm sure that my subsequent move into medical broadcasting came from a deep conviction that the best way for you to prevent medical mistakes and get the most out of your medical care is for you to have enough information to participate in that care.

While some people might think that knowledge about how to tell if your doctor is competent or how to examine yourself is dangerous, I firmly believe that such knowledge is both your right and your key to a longer, healthier life.

That's what *Smart Medicine* is all about. It's simply the best medical care for your money, brought about by your understanding and your participation.

Smart Medicine cannot and should not be used to replace your doctor, but it will help you to communicate with him and provide you with enough information to know which questions to ask and where and how to go about getting answers. At a time when medical costs are skyrocketing and medical technology is creating new tests and treatments every day, you'll learn to use your doctor as a *resource,* rather than as the *only source* of medical information. You'll visit the doctor less often and have fewer tests, but each visit you do make and each test you do take will be more fruitful.

You'll save money while promoting your health, and I sincerely believe that the mistake that may have cost Jay Ira his life will prevent other mistakes and lead to many positive, good things in the lives of other people.

ONE

You Can Prevent Medical Mistakes

Eight-year-old Annie Taylor was rushed to the emergency room after waking up at 2:30 A.M. with a belly pain that wouldn't go away. Tall people wearing green pajamas and masks, strange smells, bright lights— all this was seen through the distorting lenses of pain, fear, and simple exhaustion, at a time when little girls are usually asleep.

The doctor examined Annie and told her mother the child needed to be admitted to the hospital in order "to rule out appendicitis." Her mother reluctantly agreed. The next morning Annie was operated on, but by then it was daytime and things didn't seem so frightening. She did fine. She has the scar to prove it.

However, she didn't have appendicitis.

When Annie visited the doctor for a follow-up exam the next week, he told her mother that the lab reports on the tissue he removed during surgery showed that Annie had mesenteric lymphadenitis, a condition that sometimes goes away on its own in forty-eight hours.

"Do you mean to tell me that she didn't need surgery after all?" her mother exclaimed.

Annie had been misdiagnosed; the problem turned out to be something different than what the doctor thought. It happens more often than any of us would like to think.

Most people believe that doctors are unerring sleuths, faultless detectives who sift through the most confusing symptoms to arrive at the correct diagnosis for what ails us. That sort of faith had its place a hundred years ago, when all your doctor had to help him practice medicine were his hands and his intuition. It even made sense a few decades ago, when many people thought that all you needed to stay healthy were directions to the doctor's office for your yearly physical and a phone number to call in case of emergency. However, the practice of medicine has changed in some major ways during the past twenty years.

Many things that were the stuff of science fiction when we were kids are reality today. You can have your blood cholesterol checked in just thirty seconds. You can lie down beside a giant magnet and have your internal organs examined without painful injections or exposure to dangerous radiation. Technology has vastly improved medical care, but it has also created a complex new language and a dizzying array of choices that can confuse you and cost you time, money—even your life. Your doctor may have to study twice as hard as he did in medical school, just to keep up. The only way to protect your health and take advantage of the new opportunities is to learn the language and get involved.

What follows is an explanation of Annie's case and nine other examples of common medical mistakes. The list is not official: no medical organization publishes such a grouping. It's been compiled from extensive canvassing of doctors and insurance companies, as well as from my own experience in the practice of internal and emergency medicine and as a member of the medical media. It is by no means a complete list, but it covers a representative variety of conditions.

If you experience symptoms similar to the ones described, don't panic. Very few people with these problems go on to develop serious complications, and you'll be able to protect your own health by reading the stories carefully and following the guidelines provided. Each case is a fictionalized composite, a worst-case scenario which will explain why the mistake occurred and help you to understand how *Smart Medicine* will help you to prevent something similar from happening to you.

ANNIE'S "APPENDICITIS": A NECESSARY MISTAKE?

The doctor may have been right in this case. A more thorough understanding of appendicitis and why its diagnosis is difficult will explain why this may have been one of the few "necessary" mistakes.

Appendicitis means inflammation and/or infection of the appendix, a vestigial (present in our ancestors but of no real known use to us) outpouching of the intestine. The inflammation may be caused by a piece of food lodging in the appendix, or by the appendix twisting on itself.

Pain in the right lower part of the abdomen is sometimes, but not always the first symptom. You may also lose your appetite, or feel nauseated and vomit. Constipation is not unusual, and about 10 percent of patients have diarrhea. Fever is common, but it is not essential for diagnosis.

Appendicitis is difficult to diagnose because we can't see the inside of the appendix. We therefore rely on symptoms, lab tests, and x-rays. Annie had a fever and belly pain and was admitted for observation. When the pain didn't go away, surgery was performed.

The doctor chose to make his error on the side of safety. He could have waited longer while he considered other possibilities, but if Annie did have appendicitis, her appendix might have burst and the danger would have been even greater than that associated with surgery. The doctor made what we call a "rule-out" or tentative diagnosis, choosing the safest route because he wanted to save Annie's life.

Many surgeons claim that such "rule-outs" are necessary to save all patients with real appendicitis. They may be right, but if you develop pain in your abdomen, ask the following questions of yourself and the doctor:

- Where is the pain? Appendicitis doesn't always cause pain, but when it does, it most often hurts over the right lower part of your abdomen. It can hurt elsewhere, but this location makes it more likely that appendicitis is at the root of the pain.
- Has there been an associated fever or loss of appetite? Both of these findings increase the likelihood of appendicitis.
- Have x-rays and lab tests been done? They can help your doctor to narrow down the diagnosis.
- If surgery is being planned, is there time for repeat tests? There may not be, but you should ask. Repeat tests sometimes show that appendicitis is not the problem, after all.
- Has the doctor considered other possibilities such as gallbladder, liver, ulcer, or ovarian problems?
- Whatever your symptoms, remember: if you're confused or unsure, you're entitled to a second opinion.

Annie's misdiagnosis may have been necessary, but her mother would have felt a lot safer if she had known what you will learn in Chapter Fourteen about blood tests and in Chapter Three about physical exams and abdominal pain. She'd have been able to participate in the decision and protect both her child's health and her own peace of mind.

The same sorts of things apply to all of the following situations as well, where real mistakes were made.

MITRAL VALVE PROLAPSE: WHEN STRESS IS NOT THE CAUSE OF THE HEART PROBLEM

For several nights in a row, Ellen—a thin, healthy, 30-year-old house-wife—was awakened by "palpitations." Her heart would start beating very fast and pound so hard that she could hear it. She felt light-headed, and thought she felt her heart skipping beats. She visited her doctor and described her symptoms. During the exam, she related a history of being under severe emotional stress and having been on a crash diet.

After the physical, an electrocardiogram, and lab tests, Ellen's doctor informed her that she was physically well. He confirmed her suspicion that she was suffering from anxiety, told her to "take it easy," and pre-scribed a mild tranquilizer to get her through the rough times.

After a few weeks the symptoms disappeared, and Ellen felt so much better that she took up a new hobby—running. One day, however, while Ellen was jogging with her husband, she suddenly collapsed to the ground and lost consciousness. Her husband performed CPR and saved her life while another jogger called an ambulance.

At the hospital, the doctor said that she had experienced ventricular fibrillation, an abnormal rhythm of the heart which often proves fatal. Ellen was lucky, but she needed a work-up to determine why the problem had occurred and what could be done to keep it from occurring again.

After a few simple tests revealed that Ellen had mitral valve prolapse, the doctor explained the situation to her husband: "It's a congenital condition that usually causes no problems at all. Most people who have it live full, normal lives and never require treatment. But a very small percentage of them are at risk to develop this life-threatening heart rhythm. We can tell who those people are with these tests, and we can almost always prevent the problem from occurring. She should have had this work-up much sooner."

"Prolapse" means to fall or slip out of place. Mitral valve prolapse, which affects nearly 10 percent of the population, occurs when one part of the heart's mitral valve slips or drops slightly below its normal position.

The condition may occasionally cause pain or what most people call palpitations: fast, pounding heartbeats. Often, however, it causes no symptoms at all. It can sometimes be detected by a stethoscope. An expert might hear an extra click or murmur in the heart as blood rushes past the prolapse, but it may not be heard by the inexperienced ear.

Ellen's doctor may have missed the correct diagnosis for a number of reasons. Ellen may not have had an extra sound in her heart, or he might have lacked the experience to hear it. Also, the condition rarely produces changes on cardiograms or regular chest x-rays, and it never produces changes in laboratory tests, so the fact that those were normal in Ellen's case couldn't help. Newer technology such as the ambulatory cardiogram, which can pick up silent arrhythmias (see page 96), and the echocardiogram, which can diagnose the prolapse through the use of sound waves (see page 172) have facilitated diagnosis. Ellen's doctor should have suspected prolapse and investigated further. Her symptoms, sex, and body type should at least have suggested the possibility to him.

Ellen did well, she's on medication to prevent the abnormal rhythm, and she's had no other episodes of sudden loss of consciousness. However, the one near fatal event could have been prevented if she had known what you know now.

If you develop symptoms like Ellen's, ask your doctor the following questions to make sure the diagnosis has taken all possibilities into account:

- Do you hear an extra sound or murmur in my heart?
- Is it possible I have prolapse?
- Is an ambulatory cardiogram or an echocardiogram necessary?

If you have mitral valve prolapse, don't panic. Remember that most people with the condition don't develop problems and never require treatment. Your doctor can decide what, if anything, to do for you by performing these simple tests. It's better to be safe than sorry.

The mistake that nearly cost Ellen her life could have been prevented by a doctor who was more educated about current diagnostic tests, or was more aware of his own limitations. Ellen might have helped by being more informed and insisting on more tests.

You'll learn that one of the most important rules of Smart Medicine is to listen when your body tries to tell you that something's wrong. When it produces symptoms that your doctor fails to diagnose, don't hesitate to seek a second, or even a third, opinion.

In Chapter Two you'll learn how to determine if your doctor is competent, in Appendix One you'll learn how to choose a good doctor, and in Chapter Seven you'll learn about the heart tests that could help you to prevent this type of mistake from happening to you.

IS IT OR ISN'T IT STREP THROAT?

"Strep throat" specifically means your throat is infected with the bacteria called streptococcus. A variety of other bacteria and viruses can cause very similar symptoms. The only way to make an exact diagnosis is to touch the back of the throat with a cotton swab, grow the cells thus collected in a culture for two days, and examine it under a microscope. Many people do not get this test performed and either receive antibiotics inappropriately or don't receive them when they should have. Both practices could prove dangerous, as the following stories illustrate.

Carl Michaels saw the doctor for his fourth sore throat in as many months. The doctor thought it might be an irritation related to the change of seasons and not an infection, but Carl insisted on taking antibiotics. The doctor was rushed for time, and he wanted to keep Carl as a patient, so he prescribed penicillin—without taking a culture.

Unfortunately, Carl awoke three days later with a severe rash covering his entire body—he was allergic to penicillin and didn't know it. Within hours, he began wheezing, and nearly died when the allergy hit his lungs.

Mary Cobb took her son, Johnny, to the doctor for a severe sore throat. He had no fever and seemed otherwise well, so the doctor chose not to treat him with antibiotics. "We'll wait and see," he said.

As it turns out, Johnny did have strep, and he developed rheumatic fever, which ended up damaging one of his heart valves.

In order to prevent either of these things from happening to you, make sure of the following whenever you visit the doctor for a sore throat:

- Ask for a culture, whether or not the doctor plans to prescribe antibiotics.
- Since rheumatic fever can follow a strep throat in children, it may be appropriate to give them antibiotics before the results are known in order to prevent this serious consequence.
- Since rheumatic fever is unlikely in adults and allergic reactions are more common, it may be appropriate to withhold antibiotics from them until results are known.
- Do not insist on antibiotics.
- Tell the doctor if you're allergic to any medications.

Johnny's mother and Carl both held misconceptions about throat infections and the use of antibiotics—and both doctors showed some of the warning signs of incompetence that are discussed in Chapter Two.

Aside from learning how to choose a good doctor, you'll be able to protect yourself from these kinds of mistakes with the information you'll find on throat cultures in Chapter Twelve and on how to take your medicine in Chapter Four.

THE WRONG WAY TO TREAT A SEXUALLY
TRANSMITTED DISEASE

Urethritis means inflammation of the urethra, which is the tube that leads from the bladder to the outside. Many different organisms can cause the problem, but an exact diagnosis is necessary, because each organism requires a specific treatment.

Jennie, a healthy 32-year-old, was told by her boyfriend Philip that he had urethritis. Their doctor had made the diagnosis by examining a sample of discharge from his urethra. He then suggested that both Philip and Jennie take antibiotics—even though Jennie didn't have any symptoms. The doctor explained that many women with urethritis didn't have symptoms, but if it were left untreated, it could scar her fallopian tubes and lead to infertility. The doctor was right about that, but unfortunately wrong about the antibiotic he chose.

Jennie and Philip had urethritis caused by chlamydia, an organism larger than a virus but smaller than most bacteria. "Chlamydia" urethritis is the most common venereal disease in this country, affecting nearly four million people. It's easy to treat, but the antibiotic Jennie and Philip received doesn't have much impact on it. Philip's symptoms disappeared (as they often do on their own), but he wound up still mildly infected and passed the infection back to Jennie, who passed it back to him. It ping-ponged back and forth until it caused enough damage to Jennie's fallopian tubes to result in a tubal pregnancy—and she nearly died.

The doctor knew Philip had urethritis, but he didn't order the specific culture that would test for chlamydia. The organism is usually not visible under a regular microscope, so it's not surprising that it was missed. But the doctor should have known about the new, specific test.

Once the correct diagnosis was made, treatment would have been straightforward. Tetracycline or an appropriate alternative would cure the problem.

If you're told by your partner that you've been exposed to any form of urethritis, make sure you ask the following questions:

- Has a culture been taken of the urethra? This is more accurate in men than it is in women, but it increases the chances of a specific diagnosis.
- Is chlamydia being considered and has the specific test been ordered?
- Has a microscopic examination been performed on the culture? This may help rule out chlamydia.

Regarding sexually transmitted diseases (STD's) in general:

- If you've been diagnosed as having one STD, make sure the doctor checks for the others as well. They often coexist, and you wouldn't want to miss them.
- You should be tested and treated if a partner has an STD, even if you have no symptoms.

One way to practice Smart Medicine is to make sure you don't ignore these diseases. Although symptoms can be absent or disappear after a short time, the disease can develop into something more serious. Chapter Fifteen explains the diagnosis and the treatment of all the STD's. That knowledge may alleviate your fears and help you to prevent a dangerous medical mistake.

ENDOMETRIOSIS AND TUBAL PREGNANCY

When Susan came to the doctor with severe pains in her pelvis that came and went at irregular intervals during her period, he quickly guessed that she had a condition called endometriosis. He started her on medication and told her to return in two weeks.

By the time of her return visit, however, the pain was worse, and she had a fever. The doctor became concerned and performed an ultrasound of Susan's pelvis and a laparoscopy. For this minor surgical procedure he made an incision in her belly button and inserted a tube with a microscope on it in order to examine the inside of her abdomen. She turned out to have a "tubal pregnancy" which he removed in the nick of time.

Tubal pregnancies occur when an embryo lodges in one of a woman's fallopian tubes. They are often painful and can get infected and cause a fever. In the most serious cases, they burst and become life-threatening.

Endometriosis is a fairly common condition where, for unknown reasons, uterine tissue begins to grow in other parts of the abdomen.

It is often a diagnosis of exclusion—made after other problems are ruled out—because it can be positively confirmed only by looking at the actual tissue, which requires a surgical procedure such as a laparoscopy.

For that reason, it is occasionally appropriate to treat presumptively, as Susan's doctor did—as long as he is willing to reconsider if the treatment fails. Had he stuck to the original diagnosis, the consequences could have been serious.

You can help out in this case. If you have pelvic pain and are told you have endometriosis, consider the following questions:

- Does the pain change with your period? Endometrial tissue contracts in response to hormonal stimulation, so the pain will change as the month progresses. Record when you feel the pain, what times during the month it's absent, and when it gets worse. You should also notice whether you have any other symptoms such as fever, discharge, or abnormal bleeding.
- Is it possible that you're pregnant? The doctor should run the test, since it's often positive in tubal pregnancies.
- Are other possibilities being considered? Infections, an ovarian cyst, and a tubal pregnancy have to be ruled out.
- Do you need an ultrasound test, or other more elaborate tests such as laparoscopy?

Endometriosis and tubal pregnancies can both cause infertility or more serious problems if they are missed.

In Chapters Eight, Ten, and Twelve you'll find information about the medical tests that can help your doctor to diagnose these disorders and prevent these medical mistakes.

HIATAL HERNIA

John was a slightly overweight 40-year-old man when he noticed sharp pain in the upper portion of his stomach. He said that he sometimes felt "bloated" and nauseated soon after eating. His family doctor examined him and, without taking tests, suggested that he had a hiatal hernia. John was relieved and began taking the antacids the doctor prescribed. Because he thought the problem was minor, he didn't call for a repeat visit when the symptoms got worse.

Unfortunately, he had an ulcer, which bled, and nearly cost him his life.

The word "hernia" refers to the protrusion of an organ or tissue through an abnormal opening. A hiatal hernia means that a small portion of the stomach pushes up through an opening in the diaphragm called the hiatus. There's a sphincter between the esophagus and the stomach that acts like a turnstile, making sure that food can pass down into the stomach, but not back up into the esophagus. When you have a hiatal hernia, the herniation may weaken the sphincter, allowing backwash of foods and acid, which then irritate the esophagus and cause the symptoms.

An ulcer is a crater, either in the lining of your stomach or in the duodenum, the first portion of the intestine. The symptoms of ulcer, hiatal hernia, and stomach cancer can all be similar.

The conditions may be misdiagnosed by doctors and patients alike who rely only on symptoms and ignore the more elaborate and disease-specific tests that are necessary to make an exact diagnosis. A "barium swallow," where you swallow a chalklike substance that shows up on an x-ray, can detect an ulcer or cancer. Another useful technique is "endoscopy," in which you swallow a tube with a microscope at its tip so the doctor can examine the inner lining of your esophagus and stomach.

If you develop symptoms of bloating early after a meal, burning sensations in your stomach, and/or nausea on a regular basis, make sure you do the following:

- Keep a journal of your pain and tell the doctor whether eating worsens or alleviates your symptoms. Food may lessen an ulcer's pain.
- Ask if any specific tests are needed. A chest x-ray may help, but the only way to rule out stomach cancer or an ulcer is with the barium swallow or the endoscopy.
- If you're put on a bland diet and antacids or medications for a trial period, keep your follow-up appointments and insist on a new evaluation if the symptoms worsen. Microscopic stomach cancers may be found in ulcers that fail to heal.

This medical mistake occurred because of a combination of poor patient-doctor communication and a poorly informed patient. The doctor should have considered more specific tests, and he should have discussed the possibilities with John and advised him about follow-up visits. John should have insisted on a reevaluation when his symptoms got worse.

You'll find the Smart Medicine approach to these problems in Chapter Eleven, where endoscopic exams of the gastrointestinal tract are discussed, and in Chapter Seventeen, where the home medical test for blood in the stool is reviewed.

WHEN TO TAKE THE "FLU" SERIOUSLY

Mary is a healthy 30-year-old housewife who went to the doctor complaining of tiredness and aching muscles. After a lengthy examination, the doctor told her that she had a "viral flu"; he prescribed fluids and aspirin, and suggested she get plenty of rest.

Two days later Mary phoned again, saying she was now feeling so weak that she couldn't get out of bed. The doctor asked if she had a fever, and when she said no, he counseled her not to worry. "Continue taking the aspirins and fluids," he said.

But the next morning Mary couldn't move at all, and she could barely breathe. She was rushed to the hospital by ambulance and put on life-support devices. Doctors told her husband that she had developed

"Guillain-Barré syndrome," a rare but life-threatening complication of the flu that causes temporary paralysis. If she hadn't gotten to the hospital when she did, she would have stopped breathing and died.

Most patients with Guillain-Barré who reach the hospital before the paralysis hits their breathing muscles survive. Mary was lucky enough to recover completely and a year later she's doing fine.

Your participation is critical. If you develop vague symptoms and are told you have a flu or a viral infection, make sure to do the following:

- Insist on a return visit if the symptoms worsen or don't subside within forty-eight hours.
- Ask your doctor if your blood test confirms his suspicions of a viral infection.

Viruses are smaller than bacteria, and might be more difficult to diagnose, but a decreased white blood count (see Chapter Fourteen), along with an increase in cells called lymphocytes, makes the diagnosis of viral infection more likely. In some serious cases, specific tests for the virus can be begun—they take days to weeks to complete—but the diagnosis may be crucial if a complication sets in.

The treatment Mary's doctor prescribed was probably appropriate initially. But a "flu" that doesn't go away or progresses to other symptoms needs further evaluation. The problem may turn out to be a complication, like Guillain-Barré, or a completely different type of infection, such as bacterial meningitis, which can start out with the same vague symptoms as a viral flu.

The exact diagnosis may not have been possible on a return visit, but the doctor would have become more aware of how serious Mary's problem was, and he might have hospitalized her sooner. As it was, she got there with little time to spare.

One of your most important roles in the promotion of your own health is to seek a reexamination or a second opinion whenever your symptoms worsen or fail to respond to a prescribed treatment. You'll learn how to ensure that you receive and participate in that kind of Smart Medicine throughout this book.

That particular mistake could have been prevented by two small doses of Smart Medicine: a more receptive and better-educated doctor and/or a more insistent patient. You'll read about infections and blood counts in Chapters Twelve and Fourteen, respectively.

IS IT REALLY FOOD POISONING?

Curry plus stomach pain equals Delhi-belly, right?

Burritos plus the runs equal Montezuma's revenge?

Maybe. But maybe not.

Joelle Bianco returned home from her favorite restaurant complaining of headache and muscular aches. She quickly developed severe nausea, vomiting, and diarrhea. Her doctor was out of town, so she went to see a new physician and insisted on antibiotics. He examined her, told her she had food poisoning, and prescribed the antibiotics which she'd requested.

They didn't work, but she did develop a vaginal yeast infection, which she had gotten once before while taking antibiotics. She stopped the antibiotics and took a medicine that had previously been prescribed for her husband when he had a parasitic intestinal infection.

Her vomiting and diarrhea slowly disappeared, but they returned violently two days later when she drank just one cocktail.

Joelle was eventually diagnosed as having an intestinal flu caused by a virus. Both she and the doctor had made a number of serious mistakes. The yeast infection was due to the unnecessary use of antibiotics, and the violent vomiting resulted from the inappropriate combination of alcohol and an antiparasitic medication.

Food poisoning means exactly what the name says: the problem comes directly from the food. The diagnosis, short of testing the food itself (which we rarely have the opportunity to do), often requires that one show a connection between the eating of the food and the onset of illness among a number of different people who ate the same food. Even when that is accomplished, antibiotics are rarely prescribed—unless a bacteria is identified and the symptoms fail to disappear on their own.

You can be the crucial factor in preventing these kinds of mistakes.

- Report any connection between eating and the onset of symptoms, especially if they affect a number of different people who ate with you.
- Do not take antibiotics for intestinal problems unless an expert has seen you and made a specific diagnosis of bacterial infection before prescribing them for you.
- Never, never take medications prescribed for another person or for you at a time when you had a different problem.
- Report any suspected incidents of food poisoning to your local department of health so that it can take action to prevent the spread of the disease.
- Don't mix medication and alcohol without consulting your doctor.

Joelle was guilty of insisting on antibiotics and then taking antibiotics prescribed for another person. The doctor was guilty of being inexperienced and unwilling to refuse a new and insistent patient's unreasonable demands.

It won't happen to you. You'll be able to avoid the pitfalls of seeing an incompetent doctor once you read Chapter Two, and you'll learn how to use medicines to your best advantage in Chapter Four.

WHEN THE "TINGLING" SENSATION BECOMES SOMETHING WORSE

Sharon was bending down to pick up her newborn baby when she suddenly felt a twinge in her back. When the pain wouldn't go away she called her doctor, who told her she probably had a "pinched nerve." Without seeing her, the doctor suggested bed rest and heat.

Sharon felt better that night, but awoke with shooting pains down the backs of both legs. Again she phoned the doctor who, sounding perturbed, repeated his diagnosis and his suggestion.

By the next morning, when her legs felt weak, Sharon didn't bother to call. Within hours she was barely able to move her legs at all, and had to phone for an ambulance to take her to the hospital, where extensive tests revealed that a tumor was pressing on her spinal cord. Luckily, she was operated on before irreversible damage had occurred, and her second baby is on the way.

Very few patients with back pain turn out to have spinal cord tumors, and very few people with pinched nerves go on to develop irreversible complications. But as Sharon's story illustrates, it can happen. When it does, a lack of patient understanding and a negligent doctor can combine to produce life-threatening consequences.

Pinched nerves may seem like a minor complaint, but they are dangerous when treated incompletely. Some doctors and lay people use the term as a catchall phrase for many types of vague muscular symptoms. As a result, the symptoms often are taken too lightly.

Technically, "pinched nerve" means that a nerve is being compressed, possibly causing numbness, tingling sensations, or shooting pains. If you've been in a car accident and had what most people call "whiplash," you may have experienced some of these symptoms. In those cases, the muscles may be irritated, causing them to contract and press on the nerves without actually harming them.

If, however, the nerves are pinched for too long a time, or more severely—at the spinal cord itself—by a tumor (like Sharon's) or a "herniated disc" (often called a "slipped disc" which happens when the spongy material between the vertebrae is injured and "slips" backward, pressing on spinal nerves), leaving it untreated could result in grave consequences.

Sharon's doctor was dangerously cavalier about her problem. Although her twinge after picking up the baby may have been a misleading coincidence and there was no way for the doctor to know that she had a tumor (since he hadn't examined her), the progressive symptoms should have alerted him to the possibility that something more serious was going on.

If you develop symptoms like these after an accident or other injury, or without any known cause, make sure you do the following:

- See the doctor; a phone call will not suffice.
- If your symptoms progress, insist on a repeat visit.
- If you or your doctor is unsure about the diagnosis, see a specialist (such as a neurologist) who may know more about nerves than your family doctor.
- If medicines, rest, and heat or cold don't help, ask if a more detailed evaluation is necessary.

There's no excuse for this mistake. Sharon and her doctor ignored a progressive problem that could have resulted in her being permanently paralyzed. Sharon may have been uninformed, but the inattentiveness of a doctor entrusted with her care is tantamount to incompetence.

You can avoid these errors and their resulting complications.

In Chapter Thirteen you'll read about CAT scans and MRI, which simplify the diagnosis of pinched nerves. In Chapter Three you'll learn how to examine your own nervous system for early warning signs of trouble, and in Chapter Two you'll find measures you can take to ensure that your doctor is competent and attentive.

TOXIC SHOCK SYNDROME

Toxic shock syndrome has claimed the lives of many otherwise healthy women. Tampons have been identified as a major risk factor for its development, but the disease is not always associated with tampons, it doesn't exclusively affect women, and for all we've learned about its diagnosis and treatment, it still can fool us.

Kathleen had finished her period two days before she developed fever, aches, nausea, and vomiting, so she didn't think of the possibility she had toxic shock when she called her doctor. Besides, she didn't have the rash that she had heard was the sine qua non for the diagnosis. She didn't even mention the period, or the fact that she was now using a new tampon, and a new diaphragm. Since her symptoms were so vague her doctor thought she had the "flu" and suggested she take aspirin and fluids, and see him the next day. When she did call in the middle of the night, she sounded strange and disoriented, but the doctor assumed those symptoms were a result of her high fever. He reminded her only that she had an appointment with him in the morning.

She never made it. When her mother came to pick her up in the morning, she had trouble arousing Kathleen, who was lethargic and still disoriented. Her mother became alarmed and called an ambulance to take Kathleen to the hospital, where the diagnosis of toxic shock syndrome was made in the nick of time.

Toxic shock syndrome occurs when the bacteria, *Staphylococcus aureus,* release a toxin into the bloodstream, causing fever, confusion, and, sometimes death. This bacterium lives in the vagina of many women without causing problems. But when something happens to force it into the bloodstream, the life-threatening condition can develop. The evidence that implicates tampons also reveals that the highly absorbent types are the most dangerous, probably because they're left in place for so long, and possibly because they cause tiny bruises on the cervix. Some reports suggest that diaphragms can do the same in a small percentage of women, and there have been rare cases of toxic shock that did not involve either a tampon or a diaphragm. Whatever the precipitating cause, the symptoms are usually the same.

Toxic shock syndrome begins with fever, vomiting, and diarrhea. Kathleen was correct in assuming that the rash was an important symptom, but she was mistaken about its timing. While the rash may affect the genitals, the trunk, the palms, and the soles, it often begins after the other symptoms. It is usually raised, red, itchy, or painful, and almost always goes on to "desquamate," or peel off, as the victim recovers. Sore throat and swollen eyes may also be present, and the confusion that occurs as the toxin and fever hit the nervous system is usually a serious sign.

We don't know which women have *S. aureus* as a naturally occurring organism in the vagina, and we don't know which women are at risk for developing toxic shock. Reported fatality rates range from 3 to 15 percent, but the problem is treatable with intravenously administered fluids and antibiotics if it is caught early enough.

You can prevent toxic shock syndrome. Should you get it, you can help to save your own life by recognizing its symptoms early and getting help as soon as possible.

- If you use tampons, choose the least absorbent variety that will work for you.
- Don't rely on the name: the "superabsorbent" of one brand may be less absorbent than the "regular" of another. It is hoped that the FDA will insist on uniform labeling of tampons in the near future.
- Don't make the same mistakes as Kathleen: Don't assume that you

can only get toxic shock when you're having your period, and don't wait to get the rash before seeing a doctor.

● If you do develop this constellation of symptoms (fever, rash, vomiting, and disorientation) and the doctor fails to at least consider diagnosing toxic shock, get another opinion.

Many diseases such as toxic shock syndrome are subtle and difficult to diagnose. Although the laboratory tests you'll learn about in Chapters Eight, Twelve, and Fourteen will help, they're not the only Smart Medicine you need to protect yourself against errors like this.

Kathleen's story illustrates some of the basic problems in medical practice that you'll be able to correct once you've read this book. You'll be informed and you'll know how to give a complete history (including whether or not you're using tampons—which Kathleen failed to mention). You'll make sure that your doctor is attentive when a change in your symptoms should be ringing his mind's alarm bell. You'll learn to trust your body and insist on a reevaluation or a second opinion whenever your symptoms don't improve.

These ten stories are fictionalized and they are worst-case scenarios, but they're not imaginary. Real medical mistakes occur every day, and sometimes they do result in severe, life-threatening problems. You can prevent them from happening to you by learning how to communicate with your doctor and participate in your own health care. *Smart Medicine* will empower you with enough knowledge and understanding to ensure the effectiveness of that participation.

In the following chapters and appendixes, you'll learn how to determine whether your doctor is competent and how to choose a good doctor. You'll learn how to examine your body when it's healthy and how to help your doctor detect subtle, early signs of change. You'll discover how to make medications work to your best advantage and learn how to decide which medical tests are appropriate for you and which are inappropriate or unnecessary.

As a result, you'll be able to form a healthy partnership with your doctor. You'll know when to see him and when and how to take care of problems on your own. In short, you'll practice Smart Medicine together. Your communication will ensure that you're exposed to the least amount of danger and spend the least amount of money on medical tests. When you do visit your doctor, you'll get the most out of your checkups.

You'll be able to protect your pocketbook while ensuring your good health.

TWO

How to Tell If Your Doctor Is Competent

My parents had a son before they had me. His name was Jay Ira, and they tell me that he was a healthy, beautiful baby—for about one week. He began to cough one afternoon, and my mother took him to the doctor, who diagnosed a "mild bronchitis" and began him on antibiotics. But he didn't improve. As a matter of fact, by the end of his second week of life, my mother noticed that he was having trouble breathing, and that his lips were slightly blue.

My parents made numerous phone calls to the doctor, who reassured them and told them to come to his office in the morning. By midnight, though, Jay Ira's lips were completely blue, and his breathing was becoming more and more difficult. At my mother's insistence, the doctor made a house call. He examined Jay Ira and suggested calling a "lung doctor." When the specialist arrived, he quickly examined the baby, then took the family doctor into the other room. My mother overhead them arguing. To the best of her recollection, the specialist scolded the other doctor, "One of his lungs is almost completely collapsed. How could you miss this?"

An ambulance was called, and Jay Ira was taken to the hospital. But it was too late. He died, only fourteen days after he had been born.

I wasn't there. I'm not sure that the doctor was incompetent. Hindsight is always excellent, so I don't know whether or not he had any idea of what he was doing. But I do know that my parents never questioned the doctor, not even after they buried Jay Ira. In those days, we placed doctors on pedestals, and questioning their judgment was almost unheard of. Malpractice never even entered my parents' minds.

Times have changed since then. Some people think that we now sue doctors too often, but the fact that we're willing to question their competency is a major step in the right direction. The tragedy that befell Jay Ira and my parents is much less likely to occur today—partially because we're willing to question our doctors, and participate in our own medical care.

IS YOUR DOCTOR COMPETENT?

You may not even want to ask the question. You've known your doctor for years and you have faith in him.

However, faith won't save you if the treatment is wrong or the disease is misdiagnosed. Caring and communication, for all their crucial importance, do not always translate into competence—especially today. While most of us would still like to believe that anybody with an M.D. after their name is competent and has kept their education up-to-date, that's simply not the case.

We live in a world where medical technology is developing at breakneck speed. While science offers us more opportunity to diagnose and treat disease, it also leaves more room for mistakes. You need to be sure that your doctor has kept up with the latest medical discoveries, and practices them often, with your ultimate welfare in mind.

It might be difficult for you to tell whether or not your doctor is competent, but you wouldn't want to discover a doctor's incompetence the way my parents did—when it was too late. The idea of questioning your doctor's abilities might not be pleasant, but it's necessary.

The following fictionalized accounts illustrate the dangers of going to a doctor who may make life-threatening mistakes, either through errors in judgment or lack of education.

Kara went to the doctor complaining of nausea, vomiting, and diarrhea, which had begun just after her return from a trip to another country. The doctor examined her, ran some blood tests, and diagnosed viral gastroenteritis.

Kara was insistent that she receive antibiotics "because I never seem to get better without them." The doctor gave in, not wanting to argue, and wanting to keep her as a patient. He prescribed penicillin, Tylenol 3, which contains the narcotic codeine, for her aches and pains, and an antidiarrheal medicine, which also contained a narcotic, to stop her diarrhea.

She became severely constipated from the combination of narcotics and was unable to rid her body of the infection, which was unaffected by the antibiotics; she had to be hospitalized when the infection hit her bloodstream. Kara recovered, but by the time she was released, she had developed a severe yeast infection because of the penicillin.

Susie brought her six-year-old son to the doctor early on a Monday morning. Little Ariel had complained of fever, aches, headaches, and weakness for almost three days. The doctor examined the child and correctly determined that he was suffering from a "viral flu"; he prescribed aspirin, fluids, and rest.

At first Ariel improved, but over the next few days he seemed to become even more weak and tired. By the end of the week he had become completely listless, and wouldn't eat at all. He lost consciousness early Saturday morning, was taken to the hospital by ambulance—and nearly died.

The child had developed Reye's syndrome, a potentially fatal illness that recently has been shown to be associated with the use of aspirin in children who have the flu. Had the doctor read the literature and prescribed acetominophen instead, little Ariel might never have gotten into life-threatening danger.

These stories, and Jay Ira's, illustrate a common problem in medicine: caring but incompetent physicians who make their patients' problems worse because of either incomplete education or errors in judgment.

You can prevent it from happening to you.

HOW TO TELL IF YOUR DOCTOR IS COMPETENT

Incompetence does not always come through the door announcing its presence and flying its true colors. The incompetent doctor may not be a bungling, boorish boob; he might be a sensitive, caring physician who overtreats, or is unaware of new medical knowledge and treats incorrectly. Whatever the reason, though, there are eleven signs that alert you to the presence of incompetence:

1. *He prescribes an antibiotic when he tells you you have a virus.*

   Antibiotics don't work on viruses. They can make the situation worse, and expose you to other more serious dangers.
2. *He regularly prescribes narcotics for the flu.*

   One of your doctor's functions should be to make you as comfortable as possible. But medicines this strong have side effects (as we saw with Kara), and should be saved for the times when they're truly needed.

3. *He prescribes aspirin for a young child with the flu.*

Doing something like this suggests that the doctor is not aware of the current literature and/or that he's lazy and unconcerned with the results of his treatment. All children should be treated with acetominophen rather than aspirin for the flu. Ariel survived. Others may not.

4. *He takes repeated phone calls or recurrent complaints too lightly.*

The world contains many complaining, insistent patients who are difficult to deal with. But your doctor should know you as an individual. The simple fact that you feel the need for a repeat call or a repeat visit should alert him to the fact that something serious (or other than what he originally thought) is going on.

If he ignores you, or he's inaccessible at times of need, even if it's just to calm you down and reassure you, change doctors.

5. *He regularly writes you prescriptions for new medicines without reexamining you.*

Prescriptions don't always require an office visit, but the regular practice of writing them without a reexamination may be dangerous.

First of all, he can't be sure what he's treating. As with the antibiotics and narcotics use above, the treatment could be incorrect, which could interfere with diagnoses down the line. Although it's nice if he's responsive to you over the phone and gives you a prescription for enough medicine for a known chronic condition to get you through the next few days, a change in symptoms or a need for new or more medicines should prompt him to reevaluate you as soon as possible.

6. *He keeps sloppy records, or falsifies them.*

If he loses results or charts on a regular basis and has to repeat lab tests, it could be indicative of a larger problem. If he's sloppy about your records, he's liable to be sloppy about your care. If he nonchalantly changes records (for instance, adds or crosses out findings long after the problem has passed, at a time when you're sure he couldn't remember them), you should have serious questions about his character and his ability to practice medicine.

Records can always be changed with a note explaining why they're being altered, but cross-outs should be with one line, and the original entry should remain legible. If you find out otherwise, have your doctor investigated by the state board of licensure.

7. *He does not retain confidentiality about your records.*

Your medical history and records are your business. Your doctor needs a signed consent to release them, even to a lawyer.

If you hear or discover that someone other than those intimately involved in your care (who need to know details, like your nurse, or a consultant who was called in) has learned about your medical history from your doctor without your consent, you have the right to change doctors—or sue if necessary.

8. *He does not maintain cleanliness, protocol, and sterility in his office.*

You have a right to the same privacy, consideration, cleanliness and practice you found when you first chose this doctor. A change could signify a change in his overall attitude and ability to practice.

9. *He regularly comes to work looking ill, disheveled, or intoxicated.*

You don't want to jump to any conclusions unless you're sure, but take regular note of his appearance and his manner. Has his attention span, speech, and ability to interact changed? Such an alteration could indicate personal, emotional problems or physical illness. In either case, you may want to help, but don't do so by looking the other way. Whatever the doctor's problems, they should not interfere with his ability to care for you. If they do so on a regular basis, discuss it with him, and if the situation doesn't change, get a different doctor.

10. *He constantly makes diagnostic and therapeutic mistakes.*

No one can be right all the time. In medicine especially, diagnosis and treatment are difficult, and sometimes elusive. Occasionally, trial and error are necessary, and minor mistakes have to be made in order for the proper diagnosis and treatment to be attained (see Chapter One). But if your doctor makes these mistakes on a regular basis, you should have serious doubts about his competency.

11. *The qualities for which you chose him have changed.*

Does he still explain things in lay terms, or has he reverted to "doctorese"? Is he still receptive to your questions, taking time to listen, or has he become uncommunicative and aloof? Does he remain open to your participation in your own care, and to the occasional need for second opinions? Or has he become defensive and sensitive? If these things have changed since you first met him, something serious may be going on—for him—and it could interfere with his ability to diagnose and treat you.

WHAT TO DO IF YOU SUSPECT YOUR DOCTOR IS INCOMPETENT

It's unlikely that one single sign or circumstance will enable you to decide whether or not your doctor is incompetent. However, if you watch carefully for the eleven signs of incompetence, you should be able to decide whether or not a serious question exists. If it does, discuss it with your doctor, and get others' opinions, both doctors' and lay people's.

If you're unable to shake the feeling that something is seriously wrong with the way he's practicing medicine, change doctors before it's too late. Then follow the guidelines in the appendix for choosing a good doctor. Don't hesitate to call your local medical society or the state licensing board. If you discover that other inquiries have been made, your suspicions will be confirmed. If your doctor does turn out to be incompetent, your action could save many lives.

THREE
How to Do Your Own Physical Exam and Get the Most out of Your Medical Checkup

IT'S YOUR BODY

You have a right to know how it functions, and how to keep it functioning normally. You have a need to know because you want to live as long as possible and stay as healthy as you can.

Your doctor may have years of practice, which you couldn't—and shouldn't—expect to duplicate, but no amount of medical expertise can substitute for your experience of your own body. Symptoms are its language, the only way it has of telling you if something's wrong.

If you use your eyes, ears, nose, and hands to learn how to listen, you'll be better able to help your doctor detect the most subtle abnormality, before it does harm, and while there is still time for cure. You'll know when expert medical assistance is necessary, and when and how to care for minor problems on your own. You'll see the doctor less often and need fewer medical tests, but you'll have a head start on prevention and diagnosis. You'll get more out of your medical checkups because the tests you do take and the visits you do make will be less costly and far more productive.

WHAT YOU WILL NEED

1. Your Own Physical Exam Work Sheet (see pages 62–66 at end of chapter) and a pen or pencil
2. Your eyes, ears, nose, and hands
3. An inexpensive small flashlight (or penlight if you wish), a tape measure, a scale, a watch with a second hand, and a mirror
4. A blood pressure cuff and a stethoscope purchased from a medical supply store
5. The right attitude

Many people get frightened by physical changes, and they try to deny their symptoms, hoping they will go away. That may work for ostriches, but when it comes to medical problems, it can lead to serious consequences. Many diseases that could be cured with early detection can result in irreversible damage or fatal complications when they're ignored. You need to be willing to listen when your body tries to tell you that something's wrong or you could lose a very good chance at recovery.

WHAT IS CONSIDERED "NORMAL"?

Nothing.

What's normal for one of us is not necessarily normal for someone else. Differences in heredity, environment, sex, age, and life-style make each of us medically unique.

A blood pressure of 130/80 is perfectly acceptable for a 50-year-old man, but it would never do for a newborn baby. The natural olive hue of an American Indian's skin might look strange on an individual of Scottish descent.

So, while certain *extreme* findings will always be considered "abnormal" (for example, a five-foot man who weights 600 pounds, or a blood pressure of 300/190), our main goal will be to define what is normal for you.

Your blood pressure, the color of *your* skin, and any changes that take place over time or when you feel ill will be important indicators of your own personal health.

A NOTE BEFORE WE BEGIN

This physical exam *cannot* and should not replace your family doctor or specialist. Just as he or she couldn't possibly know about changes in your body without your help, you couldn't make a diagnosis or initiate treatment without your doctor's training and experience.

Making a misdiagnosis or starting the wrong treatment yourself could have more serious consequences than if you'd never learned how to do the exam at all. Use the exam to discover and understand the earliest signs of change and to promote communication with your own doctor.

You should do your first physical when you feel completely well, free of all symptoms. It should take only thirty minutes, but you may want to allow an hour for your first time. Start in a private room, where you can partially disrobe and remain undisturbed.

Follow the sequence, ask yourself the questions listed, and record your findings clearly on the work sheet. Remember, you're trying to assist your doctor, not replace him. An accurate record will help him to compare your exams over the course of time and get a head start on diagnosis and treatment if a problem occurs.

Don't deny or ignore any findings and don't be too hard on yourself. We don't care how you compare with other people. We're only interested in what's normal for you.

Begin by standing upright in front of a mirror.
You can tell a lot about your general health simply by noticing how you stand, the look on your face, and the condition of your skin.

YOUR POSTURE

Your posture says a lot about your emotions, your attitude and your physical health. Notice how you stand, at this moment when you're feeling well. Don't consciously stand stiffly for the mirror; take note of your natural posture. Turn sideways and examine your posture in the mirror.

- Do you stand straight, with tummy tucked in? Or do you slouch, with your lower back slightly swayed and tummy pushed out?
- Note the curvature of your neck. Does it curve forward or backward? Most necks curve forward, but some curve the opposite way.
- Is your back rounded at the shoulders, or straight?
- Now turn and face the mirror. Are your shoulders equal in height, or is one lower than the other?

HOW DOES YOUR CLOTHING FIT?

Write down each of the following sizes:

Men

- Dress shirts—collar and arm length
- Sports shirt—small, medium, large, or extra large
- Your jacket and pants

Women

- Blouse size
- Skirt and/or dress size

Men and Women

- Hat and glove size
- Undergarment size

In each case, make a note of how the garment fits (snugly, tightly, or loosely). If the same clothes become tighter or looser in the future, they might be an early indication not only of weight loss or gain but of certain diseases such as thyroid, liver, and kidney disease or congestive heart failure; all of which can affect your weight and your body's water content.

Remember, we're looking for what is normal for you. If these characteristics change in the future, it may be a sign that something physical and/or emotional is going on.

YOUR FACE

Do you look alert and awake? Or drowsy?
    Do you naturally frown or smile?
    Show your teeth. Is your smile symmetrical?
    Lift your eyebrows. Do they go up equally?

YOUR SKIN

Your skin is a remarkable, wondrous envelope.

It enfolds you to protect you against the bad effects of your environment. It cools you when you're hot, and holds heat in when you're cold. It's porous, a reversible turnstile that pushes poison and waste out while allowing nutrients and vitamins in. It's your first line of defense against injury and disease.

And it is the place where a variety of bodily changes will show their very first traces.

The Color of Your Skin

No skin color is normal for everyone, because of differences in race and heritage. But if you notice changes in the color of your own skin, it could be trying to tell you something important.

● Make a note of your general skin color. Place your forearm next to a white piece of paper. Note the contrast. Now hold the paper up to your cheek.
● Do you appear pale-white, pink, olive, black, or yellow when you're well?
● On future exams, if you feel ill, reexamine your skin tone in the same way. Note any changes, and be sure to tell your doctor about them.

Moles

If you discover any moles, note their location and describe them:

● What color are they, blue, black, pink, or white?
● Are they flat or raised above the skin?
● Are their borders sharply defined or irregular?
● Do they feel dry or wet?
● Does their surface feel smooth or rough?

You won't be able to make an exact diagnosis, but a change in one of the above characteristics is far and away the most significant finding.

All moles should be examined whenever you do see the doctor, and if in the future you notice either of the following, an emergency examination should be arranged:

● A new, dark, or irregular mole that bleeds
● A change in color, feel, or size of a mole

Rashes

Skin rashes can be caused by infection, allergy, irritation, and a wide variety of other problems. If you notice a skin rash, you'll need to ask questions similar to those you asked about moles:

● What is the rash's location? Is it in one area or more than one?
● What color is it? Does it turn white when you press on it?
● Is it raised or flat?
● Is it sharply defined or irregular?

- Does it feel smooth or rough?
- If it's spreading, where did it start, in one area, on the arms and legs, or the face and trunk?
- Do you have other symptoms? Does the rash hurt or itch? Do you have fever or a sore throat?

Record your answers. They will help your doctor to diagnose the cause of the rash and decide how to treat it.

Your Skin's Moisture Content

Your body is more than 50 percent water—a number that is crucial to your health. Minor changes in water content can affect your heart, lungs, kidney, liver, and brain. Severe changes can cause life-threatening problems. For example, one of the major dangers associated with diabetic coma has to do with water content.

Luckily, changes in total water content are quickly reflected by changes in our skin. With a close examination, you'll be able to tell if you've got too much water, or too little. And you may be able to help your doctor narrow down the cause and begin treatment.

Too much water. For men and women alike, excess water can be a sign of a wide variety of disorders, thyroid, heart, kidney, and liver disease among them.

Look at the skin around your eyes, hands, feet, and genital area. These areas don't swell by accident after a sleepless night or too much wine and song. They are lined with the loosest skin on the body and often are the first places to show extra water.

Note how those areas look now, while you're well, so you can compare them in future exams. And notice if a particular other area, like the abdomen or a leg, is swollen, since these too can be early signs of illness.

Too little water. The medical term is "dehydration." It, too, can be caused by a number of different problems, but it is sometimes more difficult to notice than excess water. The "tent" test should help. Pinch a small amount of the skin on the back of your forearm between two fingers and lift it up, then let it go. It should bounce right back to its former shape. If it stays up—"tents"—it's a sign that you may be dehydrated.

If you notice any signs of too much or too little water in your body, report them to your doctor.

YOUR WEIGHT

A number of years ago I read an advertisement in a newspaper for a "miracle" pill that took the pounds off while you slept. Amazing as it seemed, you'd take it before you went to sleep at night and wake up a few pounds lighter. I wasn't surprised to learn that the firm marketing the pills was making a mint. Nor was I surprised to learn a few months later that the firm had been put out of business for misleading the public. You see, we all lose weight when we sleep . . . even dreaming burns calories.

The pill was useless, as the practice of compulsively weighing yourself every hour is useless. Our weight naturally varies from hour to hour and day to day. Normally, weight checking is necessary only once a month, unless you're on a diet or need to check it more often for a chronic medical condition. But while many people are too concerned with their weight, many others are not concerned enough. The average American is ten pounds overweight, and our risk of heart attack increases with every extra pound.

Are You Overweight? If So, How Much?

The most common tables used for determining healthy body weight and height can be misleading and difficult to use. They're based on the "average" person—the one who's ten pounds overweight—and it's often difficult to determine what your "body type" is.

For those reasons, most experts now agree that your actual scale weight is not the most important number; your "percent body fat" is. (See table on page 276.)

The most accurate ways to measure percent body fat (by use of skin calipers, electrodes, or the "water immersion test") require an expert's help, but there are three simple things you can do on your own to determine if you're at increased risk, or if an illness is affecting your weight.

1. Weigh yourself now to determine your current weight, then repeat the measurement once a month. If you choose to do so more frequently, remember that there are natural variations from day to day and week to week. If you wish to compare your weight to one of the old standard tables, do so, but only to find out whether or not your weight is in the "healthy" ballpark.

   Use the same scale, at the same time of the day, on the same surface if possible. Believe it or not, the measurement is slightly affected by surface type—you may appear to weigh more if the scale is placed on a rug than if it is placed on a wood floor.

2. Stand in front of your mirror. Do you see extra outpocketings of fat on your hips, thighs, buttocks, or abdomen? If you do, you may have too much body fat.

3. Use a tape measure to measure the circumference of your waist and then your hips.

According to the American Heart Association, the location of body fat plays a role in the risk of heart disease. A man's waist-hip ratio should be less than 1:1; a woman's less than .8:1. This means that a man's waist measurement shouldn't be larger than his hip measurement, and a woman's waist measurement should not be more than 80 percent of her hip measurement.

If your measurements exceed this guideline you may be in the "obese" category (generally defined as 20 percent or more over ideal weight). Obesity increases your health risks by putting a severe strain on the heart while adversely affecting your blood pressure and blood cholesterol.

Remember, we're looking for what's normal for you, and sudden changes are of as much concern as absolute numbers. If there is a marked, unexpected change in your weight unexplained by a change in diet or activity, your body may be telling you that something's gone awry, and you should schedule a visit to your doctor.

YOUR HEIGHT

Height, like weight, is affected by genetics, environment, diet, and exercise, but, as with weight, an unexplained change in height could mean something important. It's important to take a measurement while you are in good health.

Stand up against a flat wall and make sure your back is straight up against the wall, with both shoulders touching the wall. Take a pencil and mark the point on the wall where the back of your scalp makes contact with it.

You can either leave the mark there and compare it with marks you make in the future, or measure the height from the floor to the mark with a tape measure. Repeat the measurement once a year.

In older people, any loss of inches could be the result of osteoporosis and might indicate the need for calcium supplements or other treatment. In children, unexplained slowing or quickening of growth could be a cause for concern.

Again, we're looking for your normal measurement. Don't rely on tables for exact measurements, but use them, if you wish, to see if you (or your child) are in the right ballpark.

YOUR VITAL SIGNS

Your temperature, breathing rate, pulse, and blood pressure are your vital signs: the simplest, yet most vital reflections of the state of your general health. They're easy to measure.

Your Temperature

Have you ever been asked, "Do you have a temperature?"

The answer should have been yes . . . because all living things have a temperature. Running a *high* temperature, or a *fever,* is another story. Fever is a symptom, usually produced by an infection or by your body's reaction to infection, physical stress, or disease. Some medical problems do not cause fever, but those that do are giving your body a way to tell you that something's wrong.

Most people's regular temperature hovers around 98.6° Fahrenheit or 37.0° centigrade. This can vary by up to one degree in the course of twenty-four hours—body temperature is usually lower in the morning—and vigorous physical exercise may drive it higher. Measure your temperature each time you do your own physical exam.

Oral measurements, although they tend to be lower than rectal readings, will suffice for our purposes. Make sure to place the thermometer beneath your tongue, and keep your mouth closed for three minutes before reading the results.

Your Breathing Rate

We normally breathe at a rate of ten to eighteen breaths per minute. This may be increased by stress, anxiety, or physical illness. Watch your chest closely and count the number of breaths you take in one minute. Do this every time you do your physical exam, and jot down the results.

Your Pulse

Your pulse is usually a direct reflection of how fast your heart is beating. It, too, can be affected by stress, exercise, anxiety, medications, or physical problems. Most cardiologists feel that a healthy range for the pulse rate is between sixty and eighty beats per minute, but some athletes' pulses are even slower, and as always, there are wide variations within the "normal" range. (See table on page 275.)

Take your pulse and find out what's normal for you. Before you measure your pulse, note on your work sheet whether or not you're taking any medicines.

1. While sitting on a comfortable chair, turn your palm up and place the index and middle fingers of the opposite hand on your wrist below the thumb. Don't use your thumb to feel for a pulse since it has a pulse of its own and may confuse you.
2. Count the number of beats you feel in a fifteen-second period and multiply the number by four to get your pulse rate per minute.
3. Wait a few minutes, then repeat the measurement while standing, then while lying down, and record the results in each one of these positions.

Notice also whether the beats occur regularly and whether or not they're strong.

You can also feel for your pulse at a number of other locations on your body (see diagram on page 67). The strongest and easiest spot to feel is usually at the carotid artery, in your neck. But don't press too hard on that area; some people have a sensitive receptor in the carotid which, if pressed upon, could drop their blood pressure and make them feel faint.

In the future you'll want to compare not only the number of beats per minute, but their regularity and strength. Your pulse will be an important tool in any attempt to find and treat the cause of an illness.

Your Blood Pressure

You might be surprised to learn that the machine your doctor uses to read the numbers of your blood pressure is actually a barometer. It contains mercury, which is driven to a certain height by the air pressure pumped in with the rubber bulb the doctor holds in his hand. The pressure is then slowly reduced as he listens for sounds in your blood vessels that correspond to certain levels of barometric pressure.

Just as the machine is a real physical barometer, your own blood pressure can be used as a barometer of your health. When it's too high, it can harm your heart, kidneys, lungs, blood vessels and brain. Treatment for high blood pressure, which is often easy, can significantly reduce the risk of heart disease and stroke, you can be the crucial factor in its discovery and treatment.

If you have not yet purchased a blood pressure cuff and stethoscope, do so now, or borrow them from a friend.

1. Sit in a comfortable chair and place the cuff above your elbow and wrap it around your arm. There should be arrows that tell you whether the cuff fits. A good fit is important, since a cuff too large or too small could produce an inaccurate reading.

2. Before inflating your cuff, feel for a pulse below the cuff on the inside of your arm near the elbow. Once you find it, place the stethoscope

over that area, with the curve of the earpieces facing forward, and place the earpieces in your ears.

3. Slowly inflate the cuff to the point where the dial on the cuff reads over two hundred. If you have a family history or personal history of high blood pressure, you may want to inflate the cuff further.

4. Begin slowly deflating the cuff while holding the stethoscope over that spot on the inside of your arm where you felt the pulse.

5. Imagine your heart to be a pump, pushing blood through your blood vessels by means of its rhythmic contractions. This pumping action is the sound you listen for. The very first beat you hear, sounding like a hollow *thump,* will signal you to check the meter for a reading on your systolic pressure. Systolic pressure is the active pressure in your blood vessels (the top or first number you see in blood pressure readings). Record the number indicated on the dial when you first hear this sound.

6. Now continue to deflate the cuff until you hear one final loud sound followed by a few muffled sounds, then complete silence. The point on the meter at which the sounds change or completely stop is your diastolic, or resting pressure. Record this as well.

7. Repeat the entire sequence lying down, then standing, and record all of the numbers.

GUIDELINES FOR HOME MONITORING OF YOUR BLOOD PRESSURE

1. Refer to the chart (page 274) to find the safe range of blood pressure for your age, sex, and medical history. Remember, there is no absolutely normal blood pressure, but sudden changes or extremes can tell us when something serious is going on.

   If your numbers fall near any of the extremes, try lying down for a few minutes, then rechecking the pressure. It may return to normal. If it doesn't, tell your doctor about your findings as soon as possible.

   If your pressure is in or near the safe range, record it and watch for changes in the future.

2. You'll probably get very accurate readings if you do this first exam carefully, but make sure to have your doctor or nurse watch you take your blood pressure and confirm your accuracy the next time you see them. It takes some practice, but anyone can—and should—do it.

3. Repeat the measurements at least once a year after the age of 30, keep the record, and report your findings whenever you do see the doctor.

4. If members of your family have had high blood pressure, or you have other medical problems yourself, the measurements may need to begin sooner or be taken more frequently. Discuss that with your doctor as well.

5. If you're being treated for high blood pressure, it's a good idea to

monitor the effects of treatment at home. Most doctors encourage this practice.

6. Never stop medications because the numbers look good; those results are a reflection of successful treatment, not cure. If you stop suddenly, you might experience a "rebound" effect with your pressure going higher than before. This could have worse consequences than if you'd never monitored your blood pressure.

High blood pressure is a disease which rarely causes symptoms until it's too late. Early detection can lead to safe, easy treatment which significantly reduces the chances of heart disease and stroke. More than 50 percent of Americans with high blood pressure can be treated with exercise and a reduction in the amount of salt in their diet. Most of the others respond well to medication. Your ability to discover it before it causes harm, and to monitor the effects of treatment, can mean the difference between life and death.

YOUR HEAD-TO-TOE EXAM

You're now ready to do a systematic examination of your body.

Certain parts of the exam will require that you stand or lie down, but you can begin by sitting in front of the mirror while wearing a bathing suit or underwear.

YOUR SCALP

Feel your hair and scalp for texture, consistency, and thickness.

Do they feel dry or moist?

Are there any areas that hurt or feel oversensitive?

Are there sores, scars, or bleeding points?

Is your hair coarse or thin?

Make a note of all your findings, and compare them to those in your future exams. You should realize that everyone loses some hair over time (you'll often see it in the drain when you shower), but if it begins to come out more quickly, or in clumps, report it to your doctor.

YOUR EARS

You can't examine the insides of your ears, but you can look at the outside and record any markings, tenderness, or swelling. You can also do a rough test of your hearing:

● Listen to the ticking of a watch, using first one ear, then the other, and record any difference in the sound.

Consult the life chart (page 286) to see how often full hearing tests are necessary, and get one even sooner if you notice an unexpected change during one of your own physical exams.

YOUR NOSE

You shouldn't try to examine the inside of your nose either, but you can check for early signs of disease.

● Do you notice any sores or changes in pigment? The nose is one of the most common locations where sun-caused skin cancer first appears.

You can also test for a blockage in your breathing passage, or a deviated septum.

● Put a small mirror under your nostrils, then cover one while breathing out of the other. Then reverse the process. Check to see if the fog your breathing leaves on the mirror is equal for both nostrils, or if one side is completely blocked.

YOUR EYES

They are not only the mirrors of your soul, they are the mirrors of your physical health.

Your doctor can pick up the early signs of high blood pressure, diabetes, or liver disease by examining your eyes. You can help him to get a head start on those and many other potentially curable problems by learning how to examine them at home.

The Whites of Your Eyes

The white portions that surround of the eye the iris and the smaller darker center are called the sclerae. Like your skin, your sclerae may be among the first parts of your body to reflect disease through a change in color.

Note the color of the sclerae. Are they pure white, or do they have a gray or yellowish tinge? A change to yellow might mean an increased amount of bilirubin in your blood, which is a sign of problems with your liver, gallbladder, pancreas, or red blood cells. Report all changes to your doctor as soon as possible.

Your Conjunctiva

Conjunctivitis, or "pink eye" refers to inflammation of the conjunctiva, the thin tissues that surround and protect your eyelids and eyes.
The easiest place to examine them is on your lower lids:

● Pull the lids out gently and notice their color. Are they pink, red, pale, white, or bluish? Again, mark your findings down; you'll want to use them for comparison in the future.

If the conjunctiva become more pale, they may be telling you that your red blood cell count is low (you're anemic). If they turn blue or gray, you may not be getting enough oxygen. Bright red, inflamed conjunctiva suggest conjunctivitis, which is infectious but easy to treat if diagnosed early.

Don't try to make the specific diagnosis yourself, but call your doctor at the first sign of a change.

Your Pupils

Your pupils are the dark, central portions of your eyes. They should widen in the light and shrink in the dark. How they compare to each other in size and how they react to light provide information about the health of your eyes, brain, and nervous system.

Look in the mirror and compare one pupil to the other. notice if the dark centers are the same size. If they're unequal, make a note of it.

Such a finding could save you a great deal of concern and cost. Unequal pupil size (called "anisicoria"), may be present from birth or may come on suddenly, as a result of an injury or infection affecting either the eye or the brain. If it comes on suddenly, it needs emergency medical attention.

The Eyes Themselves (The Orbits)

● Notice the overall size and prominence of your eyes. Certain diseases, such as those of the thyroid, may cause the eyes to become large and more prominent.

● Feel around the bones of your eyes and notice whether or not they're tender. In the future, if they hurt and you develop a fever, you may have either "sinusitis" or "orbital cellulitis," both of which can be treated with antibiotics.

Your Vision

Precise measurements of your vision require special charts and machines that only your family or eye doctor has. However, you can do some things on your own to check your vision and learn how to watch for the early signs of change:

Your Night Vision Note your vision when you drive at night.
   Is it clear, or worse than during the day?
   Make a note of your answer, then be sure to notice if this changes in the future when you repeat the exam—problems with night vision can be caused by a wide variety of problems—vitamin deficiencies among them.
   Visit your doctor or an eye specialist at the first sign of change.

Your Peripheral Vision Note your "peripheral" vision, what you see out of the sides and the corners of your eyes as you look straight ahead. Sit on a couch or chair in a room that you know well. Look straight ahead at a selected point on the far wall. Notice what other objects and pieces of furniture along the sides of your vision you can still see. This, too, will need to be evaluated by a doctor if it changes in the future.

Your Far Vision
1. Find a stationary sign or an object near work or home that has printing on it.
2. Walk away from the object until the printing on it looks blurry.
3. Walk toward it and note the first spot where the printing becomes clear; measure the distance from this point to the object by counting steps or feet or finding a landmark by which you can identify the spot.
4. Record this spot as "Far vision—both eyes open" on your work sheet.
5. Now repeat the process with an index card over your left eye (Don't use your hand—the pressure from it could blur your vision without your realizing it) and mark this spot "Far vision—right eye open."
6. Finally, reverse the eyes and record the spot for "Far vision—left eye open."

Your Near Vision Hold the book about half an arm's length from your face and read the following line with one eye and then the other.

By doing this exam, you can prevent and cure eye disease.

Notice how the line looks to you now and report to your doctor if it becomes blurry or more difficult to read from the same distance during future exams.

You should not try to substitute any part of this exam for a visit to the eye doctor.

Follow the guidelines in Chapter Six and in Table Four for routine eye examinations, and seek the help of a specialist if you notice a sudden or severe change in your night, peripheral, far, or near vision.

If you develop sudden unexplained pain in an eye, especially if it's associated with a change in vision, you may be experiencing the beginnings of glaucoma. In that case an emergency visit to the doctor may be necessary.

YOUR LYMPH NODES

Your lymph nodes are like filters: they screen and catch your infections while trying to prevent them from spreading further. They are the safe harbors where your lymphocytes—white blood cells which make antibodies and try to kill foreign invaders—reside. They are often the first place when you can pick up signs of an infection or something more serious.

Look at the diagram to see where your lymph nodes are located. You may not be able to feel all of them during this first exam (certain nodes may not be large enough), but you will be able to find a few. In the future, if those few change in size or consistency, or if you discover new ones that you couldn't feel before, you may be picking up an early sign of an infection or a disease, in which case you'll increase the chances of successful treatment.

Feel each of the areas indicated with the index and middle finger of each hand. If you discover a node, try to roll it around between your thumb and forefinger and ask yourself the following questions, recording each answer:

- Is it movable or does it seem tightly attached to the underlying structure?
- Does it hurt when you touch or move it? Keep in mind that tenderness occurs only when the node is doing it's job properly, and while pain in a lymph node should be checked by a doctor, it shouldn't cause you undue concern.
- Is it soft, pliable, or rock hard? If you discover a large, hard, painless, immovable gland, something more serious may be going on, and you should have it checked out by a doctor as soon as possible.

Make a note of every gland you found, and the answers to each of the above questions. Your comparison on future exams will be invaluable. The diseases that you could pick up are curable in their early stages, but could be deadly if they went unnoticed.

YOUR NECK

Your neck has to hold your head up, and it rarely gets any rest. It's no wonder that it's the seat of tension and very often the first place that hurts when you're tired or hassled. It's easy and important to examine.

- Feel for your Adam's apple, the cartilagelike protrusion in the middle of your windpipe. It lies near your thyroid gland, and although most normal thyroids can't be felt, tumor or infection in the gland can cause the area to swell and hurt.
- Examine your neck for any unusual lumps or masses other than the lymph nodes you've already felt. If you find any, examine them as you did your lymph nodes. See if they're firm or soft, movable or not, painful or not. Then report the findings to your doctor.
- Can you move your neck freely, or is movement stiff and painful?

Repeat the exam each time you do your own physical, and make sure to let your doctor know at the first sign of any change.

YOUR MOUTH

Examine the inside of your mouth with a flashlight.

- Record the color of your gums: are they pink, red, or pale?
- Are your teeth white, yellow, gray, or stained?
- Is there any sign of bleeding?
- Note the color and consistency of your tongue. Is it smooth, rough, or irregular? Don't be alarmed if it *is* irregular. You may have "geographic tongue," a normal variant that looks like a map in an atlas.

A change in color or bleeding anywhere in the mouth could be the first sign of a curable disorder that might prove serious if it went untreated.

YOUR BREASTS

Both men and women should examine their breasts at least once a month.
Believe it or not, breast cancer does affect men, and although it's rare, it can be deadly when it goes untreated.
Remember to jot down your findings. We want to be able to compare on future exams.
Begin by examining your breasts in the mirror. First stand with your arms at your side, then clasp your hands behind your head and press your arms forward. Then, put your hands on your hips and look again.

- Is there any bleeding or pus present?
- Are the breasts equal in size and form?
- Do you notice any dimpling in the nipple?

Now raise both arms above your head. Are any of those findings now present?

Begin feeling each breast. Start at the outer portion and use three or four fingers of the opposite hand to rub the breast in a circular fashion. Systematically check each portion of the breast for lumps. Complete the standing part of the exam by pinching the nipple and noticing whether or not this produces any bleeding or discharge.

Switch hands and examine the other breast.

Finally, lie on your bed and place a towel under one shoulder to raise it, which will flatten that breast and make it easier to examine. Repeat the systematic examination of each breast using the fingers of the opposite hand.

It's a good idea to do the entire exam again while you take a shower, since the moisture often makes it easier to feel unusual lumps or swelling.

Many women naturally have lumps which change during the menstrual period. That's why it's so important for you to examine your own breasts regularly. *You* are most likely to know if a lump is new, or has changed.

If you do find a new or different lump, go through the same motions you did for the lymph nodes and the neck and ask yourself the following questions:

- Is it movable or attached and immobile?
- Is it tender or not?
- Is it firm, soft, pliable, or hard?

Then feel under your armpits to see if you can discover any lymph nodes that have changed or that you couldn't feel before.

Record all of your findings and report them to your doctor as soon as possible.

YOUR LUNGS, HEART, AND ABDOMEN

It is unlikely that you will be able to detect subtle abnormalities during your examination of these vital parts of your body, and it would be unwise for you to attempt specific diagnosis of them should you become ill. Your doctor should examine them every time he sees you for an office physical and you should call him for a reexamination any time you develop chest or abdominal pain or difficulty breathing. Still, they are *your* lungs, heart, and abdomen, and you may help your doctor to make an early diagnosis by getting to know how they look, sound, and feel when you're well.

Your Lungs

We keep referring to the body's language, how the body is constantly talking to us. Well, there's nowhere where the sounds are clearer, where the language is easier to understand, than in the lungs.

The sounds our windpipe and bronchi (extensions of the windpipe that carry oxygen into the lungs and carbon dioxide out) make when we breathe can indicate infection, allergy, heart failure, and good health.

Place a stethoscope over the top of one of your breasts—about a hand's width above your nipple—and breathe regularly through your mouth. You should easily hear the air moving in and out of your lungs.

- Does it sound clear, as if wind were moving freely over an open field?
- Or does it sound tight, as if the wind were in a tunnel, whistling and screeching? Those "wheezes" are the sounds of strain, as the airways react to asthma, allergy, or some other problem.
- Does the air sound as if it were "gurgling," traveling under water? This might indicate infection or heart failure.

Now repeat the same steps and ask the same questions while placing the stethoscope over the other breast.

Record all of your findings.

Never delay getting medical treatment for shortness of breath or other problems that may be related to the lungs, but do get to know how your lungs sound when you're healthy and report any changes you find on subsequent exams to your doctor.

Your Heart

It takes years to learn how to examine the heart, to be able to hear all of the sounds, and know what they mean. You can't make a specific diagnosis, but you can learn how your heart sounds under normal circumstances, and you may help your doctor pick up a subtle diagnosis if you notice a change on one of your own future exams.

With most people the heart lies in the middle of chest, slightly toward the left (see diagram, page 67).

Look at the skin overlying that area. Can you see any small pulsation? It's not obvious in most people, but if you do see it, place your index finger over the area and feel it.

If you don't see it, feel lightly over the entire area and see if you can find a point where the pulse is strongest. This is called your "point of maximum impulse" (your PMI). If you discover it, record on the diagram where it lies.

If the point is in a different location in the future, this information may prove invaluable to your doctor.

Place the stethoscope gently but firmly over your PMI and listen carefully. If you haven't found a PMI, place the stethoscope over the spot indicated on the diagram. You should be able to hear the gentle *lub-dub* of your heartbeat. The sounds are made by the opening and closing of your heart valves as the blood passes through them.

A heart murmur occurs when one or more of the valves leaks and the blood "whooshes" across it. Extra sounds can also develop in heart failure or other heart conditions.

It takes a trained ear to hear heart sounds. Don't be discouraged if you can't hear them all, but *do* report any new sounds or changes you hear to your doctor. If you develop chest pain or other problems that might be related to the heart or lungs, *never* delay getting medical help by stopping to do your own examination.

Your Abdomen

Your abdomen contains the lower part of your esophagus, your stomach, your intestines, your liver, your gallbladder, your spleen, and your bladder (see diagram, page 67).

Lie on your back and look at the shape and size of your abdomen.

● Is it flat or round?
● Does it look symmetrical, or is it larger on one side?

Divide the abdomen into four separate sections as follows. Draw an imaginary line from the middle of your chest to the middle of your groin, then another across your waist. Your belly button should be the point of intersection (see diagram). If you develop pain, it will be important to report to your doctor which of the sections the pain is in.

Examine each section separately.

1. Look at the section and describe the shape and size as you did above for the entire abdomen.
2. Listen with your stethoscope for thirty seconds to a minute.
   You will probably hear some tinkling sounds. These are the normal sounds of the bowel movements and they are commonly referred to as "bowel sounds."

Their presence is an important sign. Record it.

In the future, should you develop pain in the abdomen, a change in or a loss of bowel sounds could mean something important.

3. Feel the abdomen, pressing it softly and then firmly in each section.
   ● Is there any pain?
   ● If there is, does it worsen when you shake or move the abdomen?
     If pain is increased by moving or shaking, it may be a sign that the lining of the abdomen is infected or inflamed, and the problem may need emergency medical or surgical treatment.

Record all of your findings, and in the future report any changes to the doctor. If you develop abdominal pain or other symptoms that might be related to your abdomen, call your doctor and tell him what quadrant it's in and what other symptoms you have, if any.

YOUR GROIN, RECTUM, AND GENITAL AREA

These are very personal areas, and you may be embarrassed to talk about them. But you shouldn't let that interfere with your examination. They can be affected by many potentially curable diseases that could be deadly if left untreated. Make sure you have complete privacy and proceed.

Your Groin

You first examined your groin when you checked to see whether or not your lymph nodes were enlarged. Check them again at this point in the exam, then systematically feel the entire area:

● Are there any unusual lumps or swelling?
● If so, do they hurt?
● Are they movable?
● Are they firm, soft or tender?

Record your findings, and report any changes on future exams to your doctor.

Your Rectum

You should feel the external opening of your rectum once a month after getting out of the shower.

● Do you feel any unusual swelling or pain? Hemorrhoids can develop without your knowing it, and catching them early will allow easy treatment and avoid painful surgery.

- Do you notice any blood on your hand after the exam? It may be from a hemorrhoid, but it could indicate something more serious. Report it to your doctor.
- Do not attempt to examine the inside of your rectum.

Leave that to your doctor, but do see the recommendations in Chapter Six and on page 236 about rectal exams and home testing for blood in the stool, respectively.

Your Genital Exam

Self-examination of the genitals is extremely important for both men and women and should be performed at least once a month.

MEN
1. Stand in front of a mirror with your pants off.
   - Notice the size of your scrotum, the sac that holds your testicles. Is it symmetrical or is one side larger than the other? You need to know what's normal for you in order to compare in the future.
   - Gently take each one of your testicles in your hands and roll it between your fingers to examine it.
     — Are there any lumps, swellings, or areas of unusual tenderness? Testicular cancer affects otherwise healthy men in their second, third, fourth, and fifth decades of life and is completely curable if caught early enough. Report to your doctor at the very first sign of a testicular lump or swelling.
     — Are the testicles painful? Development of pain associated with fever and swelling could be a sign of an infection of the testicles or the tubes that bring semen to the testicles. The *sudden* onset of testicular pain should be considered a medical emergency, since it could be a result of a twisting of the testicles called "torsion," which can cause serious complications if not treated quickly (see page 171). Report any of these findings to your doctor immediately.
2. The penile shaft should be examined next.
   - Is there any discharge at the external opening? If so, see your doctor. The incidence of venereal disease (now often called STD's, or sexually transmitted diseases) is still at epidemic proportions, and they can cause serious, even life-threatening, problems if left untreated (see Chapter Fifteen).
   - Are there any lumps, sores, or rashes? Again, report them to your

doctor. And don't engage in any sexual interaction until a diagnosis is made.

WOMEN   Stand in front of the mirror and look at your vaginal lips.

● Are there any lumps, sores, or unusual swelling?

A swelling of one or both of the vaginal lips ("labia") could be due to a cyst or an infection that requires lancing and/or antibiotics.

● Do you notice any warts?

You can't do an internal exam, but you should check for genital warts. Lie on your bed, spread your legs, and use a hand-held mirror to examine the rectal and vaginal areas closely for these *"Condylomata accuminata."* They're either pink or colorless and they're usually raised. They can be associated with an increased risk of cervical cancer, and they *are* infectious. If you find any, see your doctor. And if you have any sexual partners, notify them, so they can have a checkup as well. Pelvic exams and Pap smears, which should be done routinely (see page 289), can pick up any subtle problems that you might miss.

A final note for both women and men: the absence of discharge, warts, or other findings does not mean that you do not have an STD. If a partner tells you that he or she has one, make sure to notify your doctor.

YOUR BACK

This is a difficult area to see, but it should be examined regularly.

Stand with your back to a large mirror and use a hand-held mirror in front of your face to view your entire back, slowly. If you have two large mirrors facing one another, that will be even better.

● Is your back symmetrical or do you lean to one side?
● Are there any spots, pigmentations, moles, or sores?

Record your findings and compare them with the results of future exams.

Report any changes in moles or any other unusual findings to your doctor as soon as possible.

YOUR ARMS AND LEGS

The arms and legs can easily be examined. Look at each of them and notice their size and shape.

● Does one arm or leg look larger than its counterpart?

If so, choose a point a number of inches above the joint on the side that looks larger and measure this area with a tape measure. Then do the same with the opposite side. Record your results, in either case. If one of these areas becomes painful, swells, or becomes red in the future, you will be able to determine whether a change has occurred. In any of those cases, call your doctor and report your findings.

Now, feel for your pulse in each one of your extremities (note diagram), and in each case record whether or not you feel it. In the future, a change or absence of any pulse may indicate a problem that needs quick medical attention.

Next, touch each of your extremities with the back of your hand to check temperature.

● Is there a difference between right and left?

Look at the color of your fingertips, toes, the back of your hands, and the front of your feet.

● Are they pink? Red? Pale?
● Is there a difference between right and left?

The two major problems that arise in the extremities are those due to injury and those that cause pain or swelling without any known injury. Your knowledge of the normal size, temperature, and color of each extremity will help your doctor to evaluate any change.

Should an injury occur, check to see that the area has not changed shape. If it is swollen and tender but otherwise normal, you might want to ice the area and elevate it on a pillow above your heart. If the area does not improve within two days, if the pain is severe, or if you notice a deformity, you need to see the doctor.

Your Nails

Your nails can provide subtle clues about the blood supply to the skin, the state of your nutrition, and the presence of potentially dangerous problems that can be treated if you catch them early enough.

Look at the color of your nails and their condition.

● Do they break or have deep ridges in them (a sign of poor nutrition or illness)?
● Are the tips of your fingers and toes pink, white, gray or blue?
— If they are pink, and you press on them, does it take more than

two seconds—or the time it takes to say "capillary refill," the measure of blood supply this tests for—to become pink again?

In the future, if you feel ill, injure yourself, or have pain in your hands or feet, these tests will help your doctor to decide whether or not something serious is going on.

Varicose Veins

The veins in your legs have one-way valves that work like little turnstiles to fight gravity: they let the blood through when it's pumped up, toward the heart. But then they shut, to prevent the blood from leaking backward. If these valves break down, the blood stays in the same spot and "pools," causing what most people call varicose veins.

Examine your lower legs to see if you have the beginnings of any varicose veins; they'll look like large, twisting and prominent blood vessels.

If you have a family history of varicose veins or are on your feet a lot, you may be more prone to develop them. If that's the case, there may be things you can do to prevent them from occurring. If you already have varicose veins, the same measures may keep them from getting worse:

- Wear support stockings while you're upright.
- Do regular calf exercises.
- Elevate your feet once you're off them.

Varicose veins are often present in an otherwise normal individual, and they're rarely dangerous. But if you notice them now, and later notice any change in their appearance or they become more painful, swollen, red, or hot, they should be seen by a doctor.

YOUR NERVOUS SYSTEM

You can be a great detective.

Although many neurological problems are complex, the nature of your nervous system often makes it possible for your doctor to locate the source of a problem within a few minutes. You won't be able to duplicate his exact diagnosis (and shouldn't try to), but you will be able to help him get a head start—and you can have fun in the process.

You'll need a helper for this, since it is difficult to examine the nervous system on your own. Choose someone who has a few minutes to spare and offer to help him or her examine his or her nervous system in return.

- Sit in front of a mirror and make faces at yourself: smile, show your teeth, then grimace, then laugh.
  — Do both sides of your mouth, your nose, your cheeks, react equally?
- Lift your eyebrows.
  — Do they go up equally?
- Stick your tongue out.
  — Does it come toward the mirror in the middle of your mouth, or does it deviate to one side?
  — Try it again to be sure, and write down your results.

The key word regarding the health of your nervous system is *symmetry*. It is not so much the strength or weakness of one area, but rather how that area compares to the opposite side of the body that's important.

- Lie down and touch each of your arms and legs with the back of your hand.
  — Is there is any difference in sensation?
- Test your strength by alternately lifting and dropping each arm and each leg.
  — Then have your helper try to bend each of your arms and legs as you try to resist him or her.

Record whether or not there is a difference between right and left. Although there may be minor differences depending on whether you are a righty or a lefty, the difference shouldn't be so great as to be apparent on either of these tests.

The final three parts of the exam may be familiar. They are some of the tests police officers ask a suspect who is suspected of driving while intoxicated to perform. But they provide far more information about a person's nervous system when he or she is rested and sober.

1. Stand with your heels and toes together. Lift both arms, with the palms up, in front of you. Have your helper place his or her arms in front and in back of you to keep you from falling. Now, close your eyes and stand this way for 5–10 seconds while your helper observes how well you maintain your balance.
   A sudden shift or loss of balance is called a "positive romberg" sign and means that there's a problem either in the cerebellum or spinal cord. Record the results, give yourself a few seconds, then perform the second part.
2. Repeat the position from part one and have your helper protect you

with his or her arms in the same way as before. Close your eyes and lean your head back. Now lift both of your arms out to your side. Touch the index finger of one hand to your nose, straighten it out to the side again, then repeat the movement with your other hand.

Finally, repeat this movement three or four times and write down whether or not you missed your nose or became dizzy.

3. Walk from one end of the room to the other as you would normally do.

Then walk heel to toe, on a precise straight line, as if you were walking a tightrope.

Repeat this while walking only on your heels, then again on your toes.

Record whether you fell, "tilted," or felt dizzy during any of the tests.

These movements simultaneously test balance, strength, and coordination.

You have now completed your first in-home physical. Repeat the entire exam once a year, the individual parts whenever they are called for, or whenever you develop symptoms in that area of your body.

Keep a good record of your findings and write down any questions you may have for your doctor.

WHEN YOU SEE THE DOCTOR, GET THE MOST OUT OF YOUR MEDICAL CHECKUP

- Bring your worksheet and questions with you.
- Tell him your findings and any changes you've noticed since the last time you saw him.
- Ask any questions you've thought of since your last visit.
- Ask him to check your technique, review your findings and demonstrate any abnormalities he finds.
- If he suggests medical tests, ask the Six Crucial Questions listed in Chapter Five, page 82, and read the section on that test before having it performed.
- If he suggests medication, make sure you are aware of the possible side effects and the expected results (see Chapter Four) and that you follow the instructions.

You now have a great deal of new information about your body. You deserve that information, but don't let it go to waste. Use it to promote communication with your doctor and improve your medical care.

Call him anytime you're confused or discover a worrisome change in the exam. Your findings and reports should make it possible for you to see him less often and have fewer medical tests, while giving you a head start on the prevention, treatment, and cure of disease. You'll save money while ensuring your health.

YOUR OWN PHYSICAL EXAM WORK SHEET

DATE:_____

YOUR POSTURE

Straight_____ Slouch_____
Curve of neck: forward:_____ backward_____
Shoulders: equal_____ one lower (which one?)_____

FACE

Alert_____ Awake_____
Frown_____ Smile_____ Symmetrical smile?_____
Eyebrows_____ Move equally?_____

CLOTHING—SIZE AND FIT

Shirt/Blouse
    Size_____ Snug? _____ Loose? _____
    Collar_____ _____ _____
    Sleeve_____ _____ _____
Jacket_____ _____ _____
Pants/Skirt_____ _____ _____
Hat_____ _____ _____
Gloves_____ _____ _____
Undergarment_____ _____ _____

YOUR SKIN

Color_____

Moles_____
    Location_____ _____ _____
    Flat or raised_____ _____ _____
    Color_____ _____ _____
    Borders sharp
      or irregular?_____ _____ _____

Dry or wet?_____   _____   _____

Smooth or rough?_____   _____   _____

Rashes:

Location_____

Color_____

Raised or flat?_____

Sharp or irregular?_____

Smooth or rough?_____

Where did it start?_____

Other symptoms_____

Your Skin's Moisture:

Your eyes puffy or dry?_____

Tent test (Does skin "tent"?)_____

YOUR WEIGHT

Pounds_____

Time measurement taken_____

Surface taken on?_____

Scale taken on?_____

Body Fat

Extra weight on   Hips?_____   Thighs?_____

Buttocks?_____   Abdomen?_____

Tape measure: Waist_____

Hips_____

Ratio_____   A man's ratio should be less than 1:1.

A woman's ratio should be less than 0.8:1.

HEIGHT_____

YOUR VITAL SIGNS

Temperature_____

Breathing Rate_____

Pulse—Are you on any medications?_____

Location?_____

Sitting?_____   Standing?_____ Lying?_____

Regular?_____   Strong or weak?_____

Blood Pressure Sitting Systolic_____ Diastolic_____
Standing Systolic_____ Diastolic_____
Lying Systolic_____ Diastolic_____

HEAD-TO-TOE

SCALP

Dry or oily?_____
Sores or moles?_____
Hair: Coarse or fine?_____ Thick or thin?_____

EARS (Ticking of watch) Left_____ Right_____ Sores?_____

NOSE—Any blockage?_____ Sores?_____
Pigment change?_____

EYES

Sclerae: Color_____
Conjunctiva (Lids): Color_____
Pupils: Equal or not?_____
Orbits: Prominent?_____Tender?_____

VISION

Night: Clear?_____
Peripheral: Clear on both sides?_____
Far: Both eyes open Distance_____
Right eye open Distance_____
Left eye open Distance_____
Near: Clear or blurry?_____

LYMPH NODES FOUND

Note their location on the chart and write here whether any are tender, hard, or immovable _____

NECK

Lumps?_____ Stiff?_____
Adam's apple: Firm?_____ Tender?_____

MOUTH

Teeth   Color?_____
Gums   Color?_____   Sores?_____   Bleeding?_____
Tongue Color?_____   Sores?_____   Bleeding?_____

BREASTS

Lumps?_____   Size_____   Moveable?_____
Tender?_____   Bleeding?_____   Discharge?_____
Dimpling of nipple?_____

LUNGS, HEART, AND ABDOMEN

Lungs

Sounds: Clear?_____
           Wheezes?_____
           Gurgling?_____

Heart

PMI   Seen?_____
       Felt?_____

Abdomen

Bowel sounds present?_____
Pain?_____ Location?_____

GROIN, RECTUM, AND GENITALS

Groin

Lymph nodes felt?_____
Lumps?_____
Sores?_____

Rectum

Hemorrhoids?_____
Blood?_____

Genitals

Lumps?_____
Sores?_____
Warts?_____
Discharge?_____

BACK

Symmetrical?_____

Sores?_____

Moles?_____

ARMS AND LEGS

Sensation equal?_____

Temperature equal?_____

Color equal?_____

Differences?_____

Nails: Break easily?_____ Ridges?_____

Varicose Veins?_____ Location_____

YOUR NERVOUS SYSTEM

Face

    Mouth symmetrical?_____

    Eyebrows symmetrical?_____

    Tongue midline?_____ R_____ L_____

    Sensation—all four extremities_____ differences_____

    Strength—equal in both arms and both legs?_____

    Romberg positive? any falls or tilts?_____

    Finger-to-nose misses_____

    Record whether you fell or tilted   Regular_____

        during any of the walking   Heel to toe_____

        exercises   Heel_____

                                    Toe_____

                                    Tightrope_____

Heart and Palpable Pulse Points

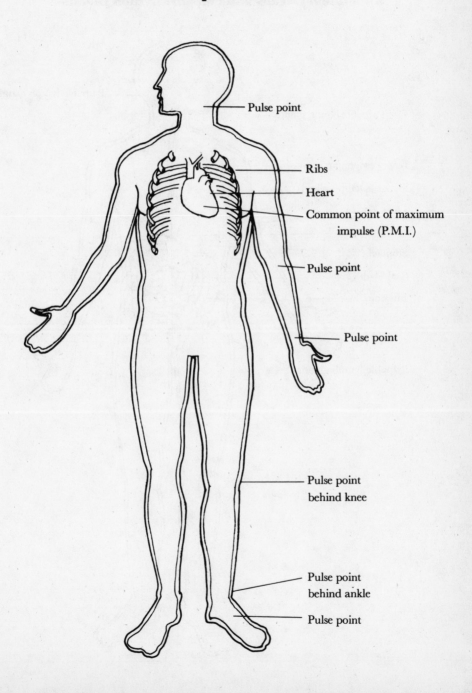

Pulse point

Ribs

Heart

Common point of maximum impulse (P.M.I.)

Pulse point

Pulse point

Pulse point behind knee

Pulse point behind ankle

Pulse point

Abdominal Organs and Palpable Lymph Glands

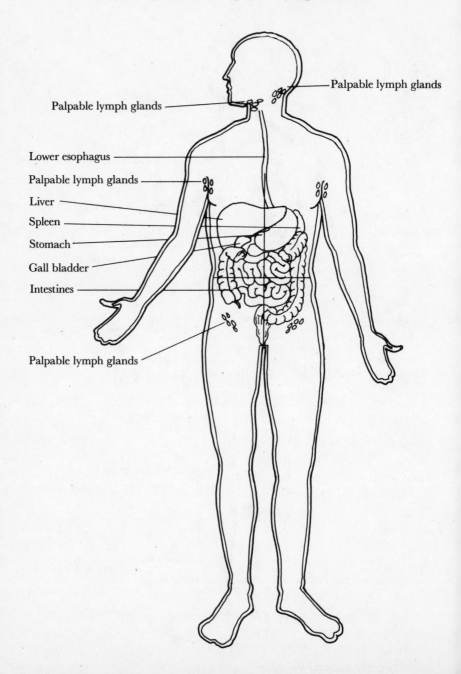

Palpable lymph glands

Palpable lymph glands

Lower esophagus

Palpable lymph glands

Liver

Spleen

Stomach

Gall bladder

Intestines

Palpable lymph glands

FOUR

How to Take
Your Medicine

Doctors in this country write more than 100 billion prescriptions every year—an average of seven prescriptions per patient. For every single medical problem there are virtually a dozen different medications, and we each spend an average of nearly $300 a year on them. Yet we often lack the information to choose among medications, to know the proper way to take them, or to prevent their dangers and side effects—as the following story illustrates.

The first thing Margaret did after she gave birth to Timmy was to ask the doctor if he had all ten fingers and all ten toes. She'd had an uneventful pregnancy, but she wanted to be sure. She'd heard all the stories about genetic defects and congenital abnormalities, and there was nothing that worried her more.

She was understandably ecstatic when the doctor showed her that Timmy was normal and beautiful: at 7 pounds, 10 ounces, the prettiest baby you'd ever want to see, with a crop of brown, curly hair and deep-blue eyes.

His first year was as happy and healthy as could be. But when his baby teeth started to come in, Margaret was shocked to discover that they were a deep, dark yellow-brown color.

She called her pediatrician, who questioned her extensively before making a diagnosis over the phone: "Timmy's teeth are that color because of the antibiotic you took while you were pregnant."

Margaret gasped as she thought back to the sixth month of her pregnancy. She had caught a mild case of bronchitis and was worried that the infection would harm her baby, so she took some tetracycline that had previously been prescribed for her husband. She didn't know that tetracycline could affect the color of a growing baby's teeth. Try as she might, she couldn't shake her feelings of guilt—or forgive herself for not checking with her doctor before taking the medication.

Margaret's story is symptomatic of a problem that many of us share. When we become ill or even just get frightened by the possibility of illness, we may be willing to try any combination of medications to feel better. Studies show that even the most intelligent people make frequent mistakes when it comes to their medication, and sometimes the mistakes cause life-threatening complications.

My own parents recently decided to take an ocean cruise. They tend to get seasick easily, so they asked their doctor to give them a prescription for something that would prevent motion sickness. He suggested the new medicinal patches that are worn behind the ear and last for two to three days.

"They're so comfortable that you'll forget you're wearing them," said the doctor.

Ominous words, as we were to find out.

One evening, Dad had a few glasses of wine with his dinner— something he rarely does. He was still wearing his ear patch, and felt good enough to take a long walk on deck before going to bed for the evening. When he reached his cabin, he was concerned that the big meal would prevent him from sleeping, so he took a sleeping pill. He drifted easily into dreams, and nearly didn't come out.

My mother awoke at three A.M. to find him wandering around the cabin "looking for the car keys." By the time she shook herself awake, she had heard enough jibberish from him to be sure that he was "having a stroke." He was complete disoriented and had no idea where he was.

Mom tried to remain calm while she summoned the ship's doctor, who, after doing a complete examination and taking a thorough history, told her that Dad had mixed too many different types of medicines.

"A little more, and we'd be calling a helicopter to take him to the hospital," said the doctor. "As it is, it will take him two or three days to recover. He'll be fine, but he should have known better."

Both he and his doctor should have known better. His doctor should have warned him about the dangers of mixing medications. And he should have thought about what he was mixing, and taken more responsibility for his own health.

My father's and Margaret's experiences are not unique. When medications are taken improperly, they may not only fail to work; they may cause serious harm. If you learn to choose and take your medicines properly, you'll minimize the dangers while ensuring the optimum result.

You don't have to memorize the characteristics and side effects of every medication and every combination of medicines in order to achieve this goal. You need only to learn a few general guidelines and a few simple rules.

WHEN A DOCTOR GIVES YOU A PRESCRIPTION, READ IT CAREFULLY

If you've ever tried to read a medical chart or a prescription, you're probably convinced that the doctor took a course in "Advanced Illegibility" at the outset. But, whatever the reason for his poor penmanship, you *must* be able to read and understand the prescription. If you can't make it out, ask the doctor or the pharmacist to read it to you.

How to Read Your Prescription

The following is a typical prescription containing commonly used abbreviations and terms.

Your Name   **Date Written**

Address

RX: Erythromycin, 250-mg. tabs   *The medicine and the dosage*
Disp: #40   *The number of pills or the amount of fluid the pharmacist is to dispense to you*
Sig 1/1 qid × 10 d   *The directions for taking the medicine*
Refill 1   *If you get a refill, you can go back without calling the doctor*

DEA No.   *Doctor's Drug Enforcement Agency identification number for prescribing narcotics and other controlled substances*

State No.   *Doctor's state license number*

                                          Doctor's signature

                                          Doctor's printed name

Many codes used in prescriptions are abbreviations of Latin words; if you learn what a few abbreviations mean, you may be surprised that you *can* decipher your doctor's prescriptions.

Rx   "recipe"; this is the prescription. "Rx" comes from mythology: it was Jupiter's sign for favorable response.

Disp   "dispense"; how much the pharmacist should give you, how many capsules or how much fluid.

Sig   "let it be labeled"; these are your specific instructions. "Sig qid" means take the medicine four times a day, and "10 d" means "for 10 days."

The amount of each unit dose is expressed as a sort of fraction; thus 1/2 means one half capsule or teaspoon.

ac   before meals

pc   after meals

hs   at bedtime

q   "every"; "qhs" means "every night at bedtime"

h   hour; "q4h" means "every four hours"

d   day; "qd" means "every day"

bid   twice in a day

tid   three times in a day

qid   four times in a day

po   by mouth

stat   at once

aa   equal amounts of each

g   gram

mg   milligram

ml   milliliter

gr   grain

Make Sure You Understand the Medicine and the Instructions Completely

1. Have the doctor clarify any illegible words.
2. Ask questions about the specific instructions.
   a. "How often should I take it?" Does four times a day mean every six hours, or four times randomly during 24 hours, or four times when you're awake? Do you have to get up at three A.M. to take one?
   These questions may seem foolish, but the answers are crucial. Some

medicines need to be taken a certain number of hours apart, and you'll need to wake up to take a dose in order to maintain a higher level of the medicine in your blood.

b. "Do I have to take the whole course of treatment?" You may feel better in two days, but if the prescription is for ten, there's usually a reason for it. In the case of some infections, ten days may be required to wipe it out, and if you cut the treatment short, the infection may come back quickly.

c. "Do I get a refill?"

d. "Should the medicine be taken with food, or should I avoid food?" Certain medications irritate the stomach unless food is taken with them. The effects of others are enhanced by eating, while some are impaired by even a small meal. You have to know the difference.

e. "What about exercise?" As with food, physical activity can enhance or impair a medicine's effect. You need to know what to do or not to do ahead of time.

f. "Are there other things I should do, or avoid? For example, do I need to stay indoors?" Some medicines make you sun-sensitive. In addition to turning Timmy's teeth brown, the tetracycline made Margaret susceptible to a severe sunburn.

3. "How soon will the medicine work?" This is an important question. Many parents spend sleepless nights and make unnecessary repeat visits to the emergency room when their child's ear infection doesn't completely clear up in twenty-four hours. Knowing when to expect results will save you anxiety and money.

4. "What should I do if it doesn't work within that period of time?" Knowing how to treat the symptoms will save pain and discomfort, and knowing when a repeat visit or a change in medication *is* necessary could save a life.

5. "What sort of side effects are possible?" Knowing ahead of time to expect nausea, a change in urine color, or some other side effect will prevent you from getting frightened unnecessarily. If any side effect becomes too uncomfortable, call your doctor and ask for an alternative prescription.

If you experience any allergic reaction, such as a rash that begins while you're taking any medication, you should stop taking the medication and call your doctor. A reaction that includes wheezing, shortness of breath, or light-headedness should make you seek emergency treatment as soon as possible.

6. "What effect will combining the medicine with other drugs have?" This may be the most important question of all. Some medicines enhance each other's action. Others affect each other in such a way that more or less of each is needed when they're taken together. If you

don't know the result of the combination, you could endanger your life. For instance, doses of alcohol and tranquilizers that are harmless in themselves can become lethal when mixed. A patient who is put on "blood thinners"—which prolong blood's "clotting time"—might hemorrhage if he takes an excessive amount of aspirin, which also interferes with clotting. Some combinations can lead to violent reactions, such as the severe nausea and vomiting that can result from combining alcohol with certain antiparasitic drugs.

In order to avoid all of these potential dangers, and make sure that you take the correct dosages when combining medicines, be specific when you get to this question. Ask the following:

a. "How will the medicines I'm already taking affect this new prescription and vice versa?"
b. "Do the dosages need to be adjusted?"
c. "Are there new and specific things I have to avoid while combining these medicines: the sun, alcohol, the birth control pill?"
d. "Are there new and specific side effects that I should expect?"

Make sure that you ask each question every time you receive a new prescription. Refer to Table Two (page 277) for further information on the effects of specific drugs when taken in combination with other drugs, or alcohol or tobacco; and when taken in the presence of another physical condition such as pregnancy.

Once You Understand the Prescription, Ask If You Can Purchase a Generic Medicine Instead of a Brand Name

A generic medicine is one which is sold by the chemical name rather than the brand or manufacturer's name. Tylenol is one brand name for the generic drug acetominophen, for instance, and Advil and Nuprin are two brand names for the generic ibuprophen.

Generic drugs are often less expensive than their brand-name varieties, and they are often equally safe and efficient. But there are some differences you should know about.

Although generic drugs have the same active ingredients as their brand-name counterparts, the process by which they're made might be slightly different, and that could alter their effects. They might be slightly more or less potent than the better-known varieties, and they might produce different side effects and dangers.

This doesn't mean that you always have to buy brand names when it comes to medications—just that you have to check each prescription individually before deciding. The following steps will ensure that you get the least expensive, most reliable medications:

1. Ask your doctor if the generic variety is suitable in your case. If it is, ask him at which pharmacies he recommends you buy them. A reputable doctor and a reliable pharmacy will usually get you the safest medications.
2. Once you find a pharmacy that both you and your doctor like, try to shop there as often as possible. Consistent relationships will help guard your safety—and you'll have a place to go if you develop any problems.
3. Ask your pharmacist which companies make his generic drugs. Ask whether he has a long-term relationship with them and if he trusts their reliability.
4. If you suspect that a generic drug is affecting you differently than a brand name did in the past—if it's not doing its job or if it causes side effects you didn't expect—stop taking the medication and call your doctor for a replacement.

HOW TO TAKE YOUR MEDICINE

Things You Should Always Do

1. Make sure your medicines are labeled properly. Make sure the labels are clear. Don't get liquid on them, and clean them off or reprint them if they get smudged.

   Keep medicines in separate bottles. Mixing different medicines in the same bottle could result in your taking the wrong medicine when it's dark or you're tired.
2. Store your medicine carefully and according to instructions. Certain medications are affected by heat, cold, light, or moisture. Improper storage could cause them to change chemically, and produce some unpleasant surprises.
3. Keep them in bottles with tamper-proof tops, out of the reach of children.
4. Follow instructions carefully. Correct timing can make the difference between a medicine's working or causing harm. For example, one that needs to be taken every four hours could lose its effect if you don't wake up in time to take it, while another may be unaffected by the missed dose.

   Individual dosage is crucial. What works for an obese man of 50 could endanger a young child's life. Be clear about the instructions, and don't hesitate to call your doctor or pharmacist if you're confused.

5. Make a list of what you take and when each medication should be taken. This will help you remember what you've taken, give your doctor a record, and provide valuable information if you become ill.

6. Pay close attention to the expiration date. An expired medicine may not only fail to produce the desired result, it may produce some very undesirable side effects. Discard all medicines as soon as they reach their expiration date.

7. Finish the entire course that has been prescribed. Even if you feel better, the full length of time may be necessary to eradicate the condition, or it may come back with more force than before.

8. Be aware of potential side effects and dangers. Such knowledge will ease your anxiety should they occur, and help you decide when a return visit or a change in medication is necessary.

9. Stop any medication at the first sign of an unexpected side effect. It could get worse if you ignore it. Call your doctor to discuss it; you may need an alternative prescription.

10. Be mindful of the effects of food, exercise, and combining medications.

Things You Should Never Do

1. Never give yourself an injection unless directed to do so by a physician. Appropriate reasons for self-injection may include diabetic shots, allergy shots, and severe life-threatening situations, such as a potentially fatal allergic reaction that requires a life-saving shot of adrenaline.

2. If you are directed to give yourself an injection, never, never use an old needle—even if *you* were the one who used it before.

   Bacteria and other sources of infection collect on needles quickly. Old or shared needles are the second leading cause of AIDS, and one of the leading causes of hepatitis and tetanus, both of which can be fatal.

3. Never take antibiotics prescribed for someone else. What happened to Margaret and Timmy was mild compared to some of the tragedies we see in the emergency room, as the following story illustrates. A young mother brought her six-month-old baby to me because he had had a fever and a stiff neck for two days. She had already started him on some antibiotics previously prescribed for an older son and had no way of knowing that her baby had meningitis and that her action might interfere with proper diagnosis.

We did a spinal tap, the removal of a small amount of fluid from the spinal cord to examine and test for infection, in an attempt to discover which bacterium was causing the meningitis so we could treat it appropriately. However, the antibiotics that his mother had given him interfered with diagnosis. They killed some of the bacteria and changed the chemical composition of his spinal fluid. The results were inconclusive, and we had to guess what to treat him with.

We chose antibiotics that normally work on childhood meningitis, but he turned out to have a rare form. A day later, he lapsed into a coma and nearly died.

Luckily, the bacterial culture, which takes two days to produce results, finally gave us the right answer, and we were able to save his life in the nick of time.

The mother's good intentions had nearly produced disastrous results, simply because she didn't know the dangers of treating one person with somebody else's antibiotics.

4. Never stop medication before the end of the prescribed length of time. You may feel better, but that's a sign of successful treatment, not of cure.

In the case of antibiotics, the medication may be killing the bacteria, but the length of time for treatment has been calculated from extensive studies. If you stop them too soon, some bacteria may survive, and the infection may return quickly.

Also, if you're taking medication for a chronic condition such as diabetes, high blood pressure, or heart disease, stopping could cause a "rebound" effect, with worse consequences than if you had never taken the medication at all.

5. Never take medicine that has expired. Whenever you buy medications or fill a prescription, make sure there's a readable expiration date printed on the label. Medication that has expired can cause serious side effects.

6. Never take a medicine that you haven't taken for a long time—even if it hasn't expired—without calling your doctor. Your condition or your medical problem might be different than when the original prescription was written. A simple phone call to make sure (your doctor may instruct you to go ahead and take it) could mean the difference between successful treatment and dangerous delay or interference with diagnosis.

7. Never take medication if the seal has been broken or if you suspect that it has been tampered with. We've all heard the tragic poisoning stories of the past few years. Don't take any chances. Return and replace any medication you're not sure of.

8. Never give aspirin to a young child with the flu. Reye's syndrome, a potentially fatal illness, has been associated with the use of aspirin in children who have the flu. Use acetaminophen instead.

9. Never take any medicine you're unsure of or whose label you can't read. A simple mistake could result in serious complications.

10. Never mix medications unless you are directed to do so by your doctor. Many medications that are safe alone can be deadly when combined with others. Anytime you need to take more than one drug or medication—including alcohol—read the instructions for each medication, and discuss the mixture with your doctor.

Scientists have been trying to develop highly effective, totally harmless medications since the beginning of time. As yet there are no magic bullets. No medicine is 100 percent safe and able to cure disease.

Penicillin and aspirin probably come closest to the ideal. They treat a wide variety of problems while producing relatively few side effects. Yet even they can cause severe, life-threatening complications.

The only way to make sure that you get the most out of your medicines while experiencing the fewest side effects is to take the responsibility yourself. Read your prescription carefully, follow all of the guidelines and refer to Table Two (page 277) whenever you buy a new medication.

FIVE

How to Tell Whether a Test Is Necessary

The practice of medicine has come a long way since Hippocrates had only his experience and intuition to guide him. Today, doctors can choose from among more than two thousand medical tests to help them diagnose and treat disease. In fact, 10 billion medical tests are done in the United States every year, at a cost of nearly $150 billion. While there's no doubt that this boom has improved medical care, our desire to know more about our bodies and our determination to practice preventive medicine may have caused the pendulum to swing too far.

In a recent survey by the American Medical Association, three out of four doctors said that they order more tests than are really necessary, and research has suggested that nearly 60 percent of "routine" blood tests ordered before an operation turn out to be useless—they have no effect on diagnosis or treatment.

You can reverse this trend. Studies have shown that your knowledge and participation can help your doctor to be more selective. However, if you don't get involved in the decisions about which medical tests to have, you're likely to suffer some of the same fates as these reported for the "average" American:

- You will undergo more than 2,500 medical tests in your lifetime.
- Many of these tests will be painful, even dangerous, but only 25 percent of them will do anything at all to enhance your medical care.
- You may spend $10,000 of your own money on medical tests that are not covered by insurance.

Because many of the new techniques are complex, and many of the guidelines for the older tests have changed, these sorts of things can happen to the most involved, health-conscious people. Here's what happened recently to one of my own closest friends.

John is 36, a former professional ball player with a beautiful wife, two kids, and a good job as an insurance agent. He thought he was in excellent physical health, but the combination of a job promotion, relocation to another city, his older child's entering school, and turning 35 led him to get a stress cardiogram (also called a treadmill test).

Though he had no symptoms and no family history of heart disease, he knew that stress cardiograms could pick up "silent" heart problems, and he'd heard that "thirty-five to forty years of age is the time to have the test done." Figuring that it would be a routine test, he didn't seek my advice.

John is a good athlete, so he got through the test without any problems. He never developed shortness of breath, dizzyness, or chest pain, and the doctor commented that his stamina was excellent, but when he received the test results from the cardiologist, the doctor expressed concern: "You had no symptoms, and your blood pressure was fine, but you had some ST changes."

"What does that mean?" John asked, quickly becoming alarmed.

"I'm not sure what it means," the doctor replied. "The changes are equivocal, but they're present."

Concerned, John began asking questions. But his anxiety and a less-than-communicative doctor combined to prevent him from getting much information.

He sought a second opinion, and the second doctor agreed that the changes were present, but "unclear." He wasn't sure whether or not they indicated the presence of definite heart disease and counseled John to take a "wait and see" attitude and have the test repeated in a year. The doctor explained that the fact that John had no symptoms or family history of heart disease made it likely that the result was "false positive." This means that while the result was positive and indicated a disorder, his heart was really normal.

Still, John was noticeably shaken. The mere possibility that he might be ill and unable to care for his family worried him. He was in a quandary about what to do. He didn't want to frighten his wife, so he kept the results to himself for almost two weeks.

The anxiety caused his work and his relationship with his family to suffer; he became irritable and short-tempered, and hardly slept at all. It was only when his wife suggested psychiatric help that he decided to tell her about the test. She was actually relieved, and suggested that he call me for advice.

I told him that there was no way to be 100 percent sure that the test was wrong, but that 10 to 25 percent of stress cardiograms yield false positives—that is, show an abnormality even though the heart is normal.

John said, "But I have to be one hundred percent sure. I have a wife and two kids to take care of. How can I be sure?"

I gave him the name of a cardiologist in his new city, one whom I knew well and trusted, and suggested he get one more opinion. Unfortunately, as I found out later, that doctor was out of town. A young doctor who was covering for him reread the results and suggested a coronary angiogram.

This test is performed by inserting a tube through a blood vessel in the arm or groin, then threading it up to the arteries that bring blood to the heart. Dye is then injected and the vessels are x-rayed to see whether they contain any blockages. The test is currently the only sure way to determine if blockage exists, but it carries a small risk factor.

Had John called me at this point, I might have suggested that he consider other tests, such as a treadmill thallium (see Chapter Seven), which are less invasive and less dangerous, or wait for the more experienced cardiologist to return.

But John was anxious and wanted to get the answer quickly. He didn't call, and says now that he just "wanted to find out for sure—once and for all." So he had the angiogram.

John's coronary arteries and heart turned out to be completely normal, but he nearly died as a result of an allergic reaction to the dye.

John's case is extreme.

Many doctors might have suggested some less risky tests or concurred with the earlier "wait and see" suggestion, and severe reactions are rare in angiograms.

However, the life-threatening event and the weeks of anxiety could have been avoided if John had known more about medical tests in general, and stress cardiograms in particular. His ignorance and the resulting dangers are not unique.

In today's technological and prevention-oriented world, the simple desire to stay healthy and prevent illness can make you the victim of doctors who can't communicate or who lack the experience to be selective about tests. In cases where you don't understand a procedure, the lack of information could paralyze you with fear and indecision. At a time when intelligent choice might be critical, you could end up being exposed to unnecessary danger and unnecessary cost. You may also be vulnerable to unscrupulous laboratories that offer "preventive" examinations and tests without mentioning whether or not the insurance company will pay for them.

You can change all that and prevent these things from happening to you. By the time you finish reading *Smart Medicine*, you'll know which tests you need on a routine basis in order to promote continued health. You'll be able to decide which are appropriate only at certain times or for certain problems, and which are overused or completely inappropriate. Should a test be suggested by a doctor or a laboratory, you'll be able to refer back to the section and the tables which follow it, in order to decide whether or not it's necessary for *you*.

GENERAL GUIDELINES FOR THE EVALUATION OF MEDICAL TESTS

In the course of deciding whether or not a test is appropriate, we'll consider a number of factors. To do this, we'll ask the Six Crucial Questions:

1. What's the purpose of the test? What do the doctors hope to learn by doing it?
2. How is the test performed?
3. Where, and by whom, should it be performed and interpreted?
4. How accurate is the test?
5. What are the dangers of doing the test?
6. Is it really necessary? If so, when?

Your final decision will be based on *all* of the answers, and the thinking behind them.

1. *What is the purpose of the test?* In general, medical tests are ordered for one or a combination of the following reasons:
   - To diagnose an illness after a symptom or problem develops. In this case, you'll need to choose the most accurate, least dangerous test that is capable of providing information that can affect your treatment. For instance, a coronary angiogram (see page 113), which is highly accurate but costly and slightly dangerous, may be appropriate if its results can lead to a change in medication or surgery. But it may be inappropriate if the doctor has told you that surgery would not be possible under any circumstances, or when medications are already controlling the problem.
   - To evaluate the results of treatment. Again, you'll want to be sure to choose the least dangerous, least expensive test which can produce the desired information.
   - To screen for illness before the symptom or problem develops. These screening tests are often appropriate, but, because they're

being done on healthy people who don't have symptoms, their value has to be weighed extra carefully against their accuracy and their dangers. For example, exercise treadmills such as the one John had may be appropriate screening tests for high-risk people (who have diabetes, high blood pressure or a personal or family history of heart disease); studies show that the chances of finding coronary artery disease in these people makes the dangers of inaccuracy worth the potential benefits. But for other people who don't have risks or symptoms, the inaccuracy (10–25% of the tests yield "false-positives" as John's did), makes the test less worthwhile, and more likely to lead to unnecessary danger and anxiety.

2. *How is the test performed?* What do you have to do to prepare? What will the experience be like? Will it be done while you sit, stand, or lie down? Does it involve injections, medicines, dyes and/or x-rays? Will it be painful? Will you need anesthesia? How long will it take?

3. *Where, and by whom, should the test be performed and interpreted?* Some tests have to be performed in a hospital by highly specialized experts. Others can easily be performed in a doctor's office, a clinic, or at home. The speed at which technology is developing makes it crucial that certain of the newer tests be performed and interpreted only by individuals who have extensive experience with them.

4. *How accurate is the test?* If a test is performed correctly, which you can ensure by having it done by an expert who has experience in performing and interpreting it, its accuracy is then measured by the percentage of false positives and false negatives it yields.

   A false positive is an abnormal result in a normal person. It reads positive, but the problem isn't really there. John's treadmill test was a false positive. A false negative is a normal result when an abnormality does indeed exist. It reads negative only because it misses the problem entirely. If John had had coronary artery disease but his treadmill test had missed it, that would have been a false negative.

   The question of accuracy is crucial in your consideration of any medical test, but you should realize that it's not the sole determinant of a test's value. For instance, an expensive, dangerous test that yields results that are unlikely to change your treatment may not be worthwhile, even if it is 95 percent accurate.

5. *What are the dangers of undergoing the test?* Pain, infection, allergic reaction, or death are all possible complications of any medical test. A recent study at the University of California at San Francisco Medical School showed that 14 percent of "invasive" tests, those that involve inserting an instrument or injecting dye, cause at least one complication. You should always consider the possibility of such dangers, but they alone

should not deter you from taking the test. Before deciding, you need to weigh the risks of doing the test against the dangers of not doing it—the dangers of missing the diagnosis.

6. *Is it really necessary?* In order to decide whether a test is necessary for you, you'll need to weigh the answers to all of the preceding five questions and consider your individual symptoms and history. We'll review how to do this for each specific test.

It sounds confusing, but you can make the entire process simple by following the guidelines below:

1. Read the section in Chapter Six that reviews the latest guidelines for necessary, "routine" tests in your age group.
2. Read the description of each of those tests in the following chapters now, or when it comes time to have the test. You'll find information that will allay your fears and make the test more fruitful.
3. Each time your doctor suggests a test other than one of those considered routine for your age group, read that specific section, then ask the Six Crucial Questions as they relate to your history and your symptoms. This way you'll be exposed to the least amount of danger while making sure you get the tests necessary for the promotion of your continued health.
4. Consider the answers to all Six Crucial Questions before making your decision. We'll discuss how to weigh their importance and how to evaluate your priorities in each separate case.
5. If you're still unsure or frightened, realize that you have the right to ask if there's any danger in waiting, or if there's any safer, easier alternative than the recommended test.
6. Remember, you are always entitled to a second, or even a third opinion.

If you do decide to have a test, there are certain things you can do to improve the chances that the results will be accurate and that the test will be as comfortable and as safe as possible.

1. Follow the preparation instructions precisely.
   - Should you or shouldn't you eat before the test? Are there any foods you have to avoid? If you're told not to eat, when should your last meal be? Making a mistake on just one of these could affect the accuracy, comfort, and potential danger of the test.
   - If medications need to be taken before the tests, take them at the exact time you are instructed.
   - Follow the instructions regarding rest and exercise as well.

2. If you have any allergies, make sure to tell the doctor. You don't want to experience a life-threatening reaction such as John did.
3. If you're on medications, tell the doctor about them. They might interfere with the test, and they might need to be stopped temporarily.
4. Find out how long the test will take and what it will involve. You'll be able to plan your time, bring something to read, and bring company, if you wish.
5. If necessary, arrange for transportation to and from the testing place.
6. Read the consent form carefully before signing it. You have the right to refuse consent or make changes on the form if you wish. If you've decided that the test is worth whatever dangers it involves, make sure no new dangers (which your doctor failed to mention) have been added to the list. If they have, discuss them with the doctor until you feel satisfied that you understand all the risks before signing.
7. If the person performing the test turns out to be someone different than you expected, question the circumstances. It's entirely possible that this person is just as qualified as the one you had chosen, but you have a right to check on his or her credentials. You can also refuse to have the test.
8. If you begin to get frightened or experience pain during the test, don't hesitate to tell the doctor about it. You may have to grin and bear it, but more likely, the doctor will be able to do something to make you more comfortable.
9. When you receive the results of your test, remember that knowing what is normal for you is more important than what is considered normal for the general population. Age, weight, medications and medical history can all affect test values and their interpretations. For example, a hematocrit (see page 195) result considered normal for a menstruating woman might be considered low for a healthy young man. Likewise, a hemoglobin (see page 195) reading of 12 might be interpreted as "normal" for you, but if your hemoglobin had been 16 on many past exams, the 12 could mean something important.

When used properly, medical tests can ease suffering, cure illness, and save lives. As you read the following chapters and consider each of the individual tests, keep in mind that your major goal should be to promote communication with your doctor, not to substitute for his expertise. If you have any questions, don't hesitate to ask them, and if you don't get satisfactory answers, don't hesitate to get a second opinion, or to find a different doctor. The medical partnership you and your doctor form will help to prevent disease and to ensure your continued health.

SIX

Routine Tests for a
Healthy Life

Gone are the days when you were advised to get a doctor's physical, blood tests, an electrocardiogram, and a chest x-ray every year. Studies show that such a test schedule rarely justifies the cost, and most experts feel that the frequency of office visits and tests should be guided by your personal medical history and symptoms rather than by the calendar.

As a result, the American Cancer Society, the American Heart Association, and the American Medical Association have all revised their guidelines for the scheduling of "routine" tests—the few examinations and procedures you do need in order to ensure your continued good health. This chapter summarizes those guidelines. Wherever they disagree, the most stringent recommendations are printed.

If you're well and have no acute of chronic medical problems, the guidelines will help to keep you well, either by preventing the onset of disease or detecting it early while there is still time for a cure. If you have certain medical problems or risk factors for certain diseased, such as symptoms or family history, you'll learn how to adjust the guidelines to fit your individual circumstances.

By getting to know your body in health, learning to communicate with your doctor, and following the recommendations for your age group, you'll get the best medical care while avoiding costly or unnecessary tests.

Read the section that applies to your age bracket first, then turn to the individual descriptions of the routine screening tests in the appropriate chapter. If your doctor suggests a test which is not considered routine for you, read the section on that test carefully and ask the Six Crucial Questions before deciding to have it done. Keep in mind that *Smart Medicine* is not meant to replace your family doctor, but to assist him in keeping you in good health. If you have any questions about the guidelines or how they pertain to you, discuss them with your doctor.

NEWBORN TO AGE 5

Doctor's physical exam
- Once a month from birth to three months.
- Every two to three months until age 2.
- One exam at ages 2, 3, 4, and 5.

Lab tests
- *Screening for genetic enzyme defects*   At birth.
- *Blood count*   Once in the first year and once at age 4.
- *Urine analysis*   Once in first year and once at age 4.
- *Other blood and urine tests*   Only as history or symptoms dictate.

Tuberculosis test   Once in first year and every one to two years thereafter. Less often if no known exposure.

Blood pressure   Once between ages 3 and 5.

Height and weight measurements   With each doctor's exam.

Vision   Once at age 3 and once at age 5.

Hearing   Depends on history. Should be checked in any child who has trouble learning.

Developmental assessment   With each doctor's exam.

AGE 6 TO 11

Doctor's physical exam   Every two years.

Lab tests   Blood count and urine analysis once in this time period.

Blood pressure   Every other year.

Height and weight measurement   At each doctor's exam.

Tuberculosis test   Every other year.

AGES 12 TO 17

Doctor's physical exam   Every other year.

Lab tests   Blood count and urine analysis once in this time period.

Blood pressure   Every other year.

Height and weight measurement   Every other year.

Tuberculosis test Every other year, depending on exposure.

Pap smear and pelvic exam Once every two to three years for sexually active girls.

Hearing and vision As symptoms dictate, but one test should have been performed by age 17 in any case.

AGE 18 TO 24

Doctor's physical exam Once during this time period.

Height and weight measurement Once, at doctor's exam.

Blood pressure Once, at doctor's exam.

Lab tests
- *Blood count* Once.
- *Urine analysis* Once.
- *Blood lipids (cholesterol and triglyceride)* Once.
- *Blood sugar* Once between 20 and 39.
- *Rubella (test for exposure to German measles)* For women, once after age 18, before pregnancy.

Tuberculosis test Every five years unless high risk, in which case every one to two years.

Electrocardiogram If you are healthy and have no history of heart disease, your first electrocardiogram should be performed at age 20.

Pap smear and pelvic exam According to the American Cancer Society, women who have been sexually active or have reached the age of 18 should have an annual Pap smear and pelvic examination until there have been three consecutive normal exams. Thereafter, they can be performed less frequently at the discretion of the physician.

Breast exam by doctor Every three years.

Self breast exam (men and women) Once a month.

Self testicular exam Once a month.

Test for syphilis (VDRL or RPR) Once after age of 18.

Cancer checkup This exam should include health counseling and examinations for cancer of the thyroid, testes, prostate, mouth, ovaries, skin, and lymph nodes.

The American Cancer Society recommends that you have one every three years between the ages of 20 and 40.

AGE 25 TO 35

Doctor's physical exam   Once at ages 25, 30, and 35.

Lab tests   *Blood count, blood lipids, blood sugar, and urine analysis* once at ages 25, 30, and 35.

Blood pressure   Every 2½ years.

Doctor's breast exam   Every three years.

Self breast exam   Once a month.

Pap smear and pelvic exam   According to the American Cancer Society, women who have been sexually active or have reached the age of 18 should have an annual Pap smear and pelvic examination until there have been three consecutive normal exams. Thereafter, they can be performed less frequently at the discretion of the physician.

Self testicular exam   Once a month.

Mammogram or equivalent breast x-ray   The American Cancer Society recommends that the baseline mammogram be done between the ages of 35 and 39, but a family or personal history of breast problems may dictate that it be done sooner.

AGE 36 TO 50

Doctor's physical exam   At 40, 45, and 50.

Lab tests   *Blood count, blood lipids, blood sugar, urine analysis* at 40, 45, and 50.

Blood pressure   Every 2½ years.

Doctor's breast exam   Once a year.

Self breast exam   Once a month.

Pap smear and pelvic exam   According to the American Cancer Society, women who have been sexually active or have reached the age of 18 should have an annual Pap smear and pelvic examination until there have been three consecutive normal exams. Thereafter, they can be performed less frequently at the discretion of the physician.

Mammogram   Every one to two years.

Rectal exam   Once a year.

Electrocardiogram   Your initial electrocardiogram should have been done at age 20. If you have no medical problems, your second one should be done at age 40.

Chest x-ray   If you have not yet had one, your first chest x-ray should be performed at age 40. Many organizations *never* suggest a "routine" chest x-ray, but a few do. Hence it's listed here, but you may want to discuss it with your doctor before having it done.

Cancer checkup   This exam, recommended by the American Cancer Society, should include health counseling and examinations for cancer of the thyroid, testes, prostate, mouth, ovaries, skin, and lymph nodes.

It is recommended once a year after the age of 40.

AGE 50 TO 60

Doctor's physical exam   Once at 55 and 60.

Lab tests   *Blood count, blood lipids, blood sugar, urine analysis* once at 55 and 60.

Blood pressure   Every 2½ years.

Doctor's breast exam   Once a year.

Self breast exam   Once a month.

Pap smear and pelvic exam   According to the American Cancer Society, women who have been sexually active or have reached the age of 18 should have an annual Pap smear and pelvic examination until there have been three consecutive normal exams. After menopause, they may be performed less frequently at the discretion of the physician.

Mammogram   Once a year

Endometrial tissue sample (uterus)   At menopause, for women at risk (see page 123).

Rectal exam   Once a year.

Test for blood in the stool   Once a year.

Proctoscopy or sigmoidoscopy   Two tests one year apart; if both are normal, then once every three to five years.

AGE 60 TO 75

Doctor's physical exam   Once every 2½ years.

Lab tests   *Blood count, blood sugar, urine analysis*   Once every 2½ years.

Blood lipids   Optional. Thinking on this test is changing; it may be indicated yearly for patients at risk, for example, those who have had bypass surgery or who have heart disease or a history of high blood lipid levels.

Blood pressure   Every 2½ years.

Doctor's breast exam   Once a year.

Self breast exam   Once a month.

Pap smear and pelvic exam   According to he American Cancer Society, women who have been sexually active or have reached the age of 18 should have an annual Pap smear and pelvic examination until there have been three consecutive normal exams. After menopause, they may be performed less frequently at the discretion of the physician.

Mammogram   Every one to two years.

Rectal exam   Once a year.

Test for Blood in the Stool   Once a year.

Proctoscopy or sigmoidoscopy   You should have begun having these tests between the ages of 50 and 60. If you didn't, you should have one annually for two years. If the results are normal, you can then cut back to once every three to five years.

Electrocardiogram   Your first electrocardiogram should have been done at age 20, the second at age 40. If you have had no medical problems, your third should be done at age 60.

OVER AGE 75

Doctor's physical exam   Once a year.

Lab tests
- *Blood count, urine analysis*   Once a year.
- *Blood sugar and blood lipids*   Depends on history and symptoms.

Blood pressure: Every year.

Doctor's breast exam   Once a year.

Self breast exam   Once a month.

Pap smear and pelvic exam   According to the American Cancer Society, women who have been sexually active or have reached the age of 18 should have an annual Pap smear and pelvic examination until there have been three consecutive normal exams. After menopause, they may be performed less frequently at the discretion of the physician.

Mammogram   Every one to two years.

Rectal exam   Once a year.

Blood in stool   Once a year.

Proctoscopy or sigmoidoscopy   If not yet begun, have one annually for two years. If results are normal, cut back to once every three to five years.

These tests are your routine screening tests. Review them regularly in this chapter or by using Table Four, beginning on page 286. They should help prevent disease or detect it early when there's still time for cure. Read the descriptions in the following chapters before having them performed. If your doctor suggests any tests that are not listed in this chapter, read the section on that test and, in each case ask our Six Crucial Questions (page 82). You'll save money by cutting down on the number of tests you might otherwise agree to, and you'll be more prepared for the tests that you and your doctor decide you do need. You'll avoid unnecessary danger and anxiety while promoting your continued health.

SEVEN

Tests for Your Heart and Blood Vessels

- One out of every three Americans has heart or blood vessel disease.
- One out of five people who die from such diseases dies before the age of 65.
- Although stroke is our third leading cause of death, early detection of high blood pressure has helped cut the stroke fatality rate in half during the past ten years.
- Nearly 50 percent of people who die from heart attacks could be saved by early diagnosis and treatment.

When you consider these facts, the recent proliferation of tests that can be used to examine your heart and blood vessels is easy to appreciate. Modern technology promises to deepen our knowledge of the causes of heart and blood vessel diseases and improve our ability to treat them. However, with that promise comes some confusion and some disadvantages.

Do you know whether or not you still need a "routine" electrocardiogram, even if you don't have chest pain? Should you have a "stress (treadmill) cardiogram"? If so, when? If you're worried about coronary artery blockage, should you have a "treadmill thallium" or one of those new-fangled tests like SPECT or PET? The variety and complexity of the new tests makes it difficult for you to understand and choose among them.

Your doctor will help. He may even decide for you. Still, there will be times when the choices seem confusing and frightening, and you may run into a doctor who isn't fully aware of all the latest options himself. Your understanding of the tests will help to ensure both your health and your peace of mind.

THE "RESTING" ELECTROCARDIOGRAM

What Is the Purpose of the Test?

The resting cardiogram is a crucial screening test for heart disease. Its main purpose is to detect abnormalities of rhythm, rate, and cardiac blood supply. It can provide other types of information as well, including abnormal fluid collection, infection, change in heart size or heart failure.

How Is the Test Performed?

As the name implies, the resting electrocardiogram is done while you rest, usually while you lie on a stretcher or a bed.

The technician or doctor will attach tiny electrodes (which cannot harm you) to your chest, arms, and legs with jelly or alcohol and suction cups, then ask you to breathe normally and lie still while the cardiograph prints your tracing.

Your heartbeat begins with an electrical impulse that usually originates in the upper portion of your heart. As this impulse moves throughout the heart, it causes the muscle to contract and the heart to pump blood.

The electrodes which have been placed on your chest and arms receive and translate this impulse onto the graph paper, where it provides direct information about your heart's rate and rhythm. Since changes in blood supply may affect heart muscles in such a way as to change these electrical impulses, your doctor may also be able to tell whether any heart cells are endangered by decreased blood flow, or whether you have had a heart attack as a result of a complete blockage of flow to one area.

The test takes about two minutes and is not at all painful. The jelly might irritate you or cause a local allergic reaction, though this is rare. Should it happen, inform the technician. The next time, a different type of jelly or alcohol can be used.

Where and by Whom Should the Test Be Performed and Interpreted?

The resting cardiogram is performed in an office, a clinic, or a hospital. It can be done by any properly trained technician.

However, it should only be interpreted by an expert such as your family doctor or, when heart disease exists and the cardiogram is confusing, a cardiologist.

How Accurate Is the Test?

According to several studies, the resting cardiogram produces "false negatives"—normal cardiograms in spite of the presence of a heart abnormality—a significant percentage of the time. However, those numbers refer to *all* heart abnormalities, including the more subtle ones that require elaborate testing for exact diagnosis. When it is used to evaluate specific heart problems, such as disturbances of resting heart rate and rhythm, heart attack, or decreased blood flow ("ischemia") the resting cardiogram is very accurate.

The rare "false positive" (abnormal finding despite a normal heart) cardiogram can usually be weeded out by an expert such as a cardiologist.

What Are the Dangers of Having the Test Done?

Aside from the rare local allergic reaction to the gel, which can be avoided by changing gels or using alcohol instead, there are no physical complications associated with this test.

Is It Really Necessary?

Yes, but not as frequently as we once thought.

It is necessary as a first-line test whenever you have problems related to the heart, such as chest pain, and as a screening test to aid in the early detection of heart disease.

According to the American Heart Association, you should have a resting cardiogram whenever you develop symptoms related to the heart. If you're well and have no symptoms or family history of heart disease, your first cardiogram should be done at age 20, your second at age 40, your third at age 60. If you have a family or personal history of heart problems, or risk factors such as high blood pressure, obesity, or diabetes, tobacco use or alcohol abuse, you may need one sooner, and you may need them more frequently.

Often, other tests such as x-rays or blood tests will be necessary to confirm the resting cardiogram's diagnosis. More elaborate tests or those done while you exercise may also be required to diagnose "silent" (producing no symptoms under resting conditions) or subtle heart problems.

THE AMBULATORY CARDIOGRAM

What Is the Purpose of the Test?

Sometimes called the Holter Monitor, the ambulatory cardiogram is used most frequently to screen for and monitor disturbances in your heart's rate and rhythm, but it can diagnose other problems as well.

Since it's a continuous recording, it may be more likely than a single isolated resting cardiogram to detect "silent" heart diseases, and more sensitive to problems that occur only when you're active. Because it can correlate activity with symptoms, it can also be used to direct and/or monitor medical treatment.

How Is the Test Performed?

The ambulatory cardiogram is a miniature electrocardiogram, performed while you go about your normal daily activities. Electrodes are attached to your chest and you wear a small, continuous recorder on your belt or carry it in your pocket as you eat, drink, exercise, work, and sleep. You're instructed to keep a fairly detailed log of your activity and symptoms (such as chest pain or shortness of breath). At the end of the test, which usually lasts twenty-four hours, the continuous electrodiagram is reviewed along with the diary you've kept.

Where and by Whom Should the Test Be Performed and Interpreted?

A technician can connect you to the monitor and instruct you as to its use, but only your doctor or a heart specialist should interpret the results.

How Accurate Is the Test?

The ambulatory cardiogram is at least as accurate as a resting cardiogram. It may produce a few more false positive results because of activity, but it will probably produce fewer false negatives.

What Are the Dangers of Having the Test Done?

None. Since you are not changing your daily activity, this test does not increase your risk.

Is It Really Necessary?

The ambulatory cardiogram is not a routine test. It is not required on a regular basis. In the following cases, however, it may be necessary and prove life-saving.

● To follow the course of treatment and guide therapy in patients with heart rhythm problems, or who wear heart pacemakers.
● For the detection of heart rhythm problems, for anyone who has a history of such problems or who develops symptoms that could be explained by rhythm or heart disturbances. These include:
— Episodes of unexplained loss of consciousness
— Episodes of palpitations or fast heartbeat
— Unexplained chest pain, shortness of breath, or other problems possibly related to the heart
— Certain cases where mitral valve prolapse has been diagnosed (see page 16), especially if the patient experiences any symptoms that can be related to heart problems

THE STRESS CARDIOGRAM

Also called the treadmill cardiogram, this test is more likely than the resting cardiogram to detect "silent" heart problems, but it may be more risky for certain people, since it involves exercise. Also, it's hard to interpret. Be sure to read this section carefully and consider the answers to all of the Six Crucial Questions before deciding to take the test.

What Is the Purpose of the Test?

More than 100,000 people who die from heart attacks each year have no prior warning of any heart problem. Many of these people have normal resting cardiograms, but they die during exertion, when the blood supply to the heart fails to satisfy the heart's needs.

The stress cardiogram tries to identify these people by exercising the heart under controlled circumstances and recording its reaction. It can also be used to evaluate how a course of medical treatment is working or to determine the extent of disease in people who are known to have heart problems.

How Is the Test Performed?

First, a resting cardiogram will be performed. The doctor or nurse may then thread an intravenous line into one of your arm veins (in case an emergency occurs and you need medication) and you will be hooked up to the same type of machine used for the resting cardiogram, so that you can exercise while your blood pressure, pulse, and cardiogram are recorded. If, for some reason, you are unable to exercise, medications may be used to stress your heart instead.

You'll be asked to exercise at different gradations or different speeds on a treadmill, or at different speeds and against different resistances on a stationary bicycle.

When you reach the point that protocol defines as "maximum exercise" or when you develop symptoms such as chest pain, your doctor will stop the test and perform a second resting cardiogram. He'll track your blood pressure, pulse, and symptoms for several minutes before and after the test in order to get a good measure of your physical response to stress.

Where and by Whom Should the Test Be Performed and Interpreted?

Either a doctor or a specially trained technician or nurse can administer your stress cardiogram. No matter who administers it, it should always be done in a setting where a doctor and medicines are available, such as a well-equipped office, clinic, or hospital, in case you develop heart problems while you are being tested. Because of the dangers of false positive and false negative results (see below), it must be interpreted only by a specialist who is experienced in the evaluation of stress cardiograms, such as a specially trained family physician or cardiologist.

How Accurate Is the Test?

Studies report that stress cardiograms performed on patients who have no symptoms of heart disease can yield anywhere from *10 to 25 percent false positive* results. This means that if you have no symptoms and decide to have a stress cardiogram, you have nearly a one in five chance of receiving an abnormal result—even if your heart is normal. If this happens, you may be subjected to dangerous tests that otherwise would have been unnecessary—as was my friend John.

The stress cardiogram is much more accurate when performed on people who *do* have symptoms and/or risk factors for heart disease, such as a strong family history of heart disease, high blood pressure, heavy tobacco use, high blood cholesterol, or diabetes. For those reasons, most experts suggest that you have a stress cardiogram only after careful consideration of your heart risk factors and your own medical history. See page 99 for the proper indications for a stress test.

What Are the Dangers of Doing the Test?

The greatest danger is that you could have a heart attack or other heart problem while doing the test.

When you exercise, you increase your pulse and blood pressure, which increases the heart's need for blood. If one or more of your coronary arteries are narrowed, they may supply your heart with enough blood when you are at rest, but not when you exercise. This is, of course, the principle of the test, since such imbalance between need and supply should cause changes on the cardiogram. In rare circumstances, the previously "silent" imbalance could result in damage to your heart and danger to your life. The chance that this can happen is small but real.

You can minimize this danger by observing the following measures:

● Make sure that the test is done properly, with slowly increasing gradations of effort and stress.
● Stop at the first sign of pain.
● Check ahead of time that a doctor and medications are readily available, should an emergency occur.

A lesser, but real danger of stress cardiograms lies in their ability to produce false negative and false positive results. If you get a false negative result, you may feel reassured, when in fact you have a condition that needs attention. If you get a false positive, you might be subjected to needless anxiety and, quite possibly, other dangerous and costly tests. You can minimize these dangers by having the test done only if it is appropriate for you and making sure that an expert performs and interprets it.

Is It Really Necessary?

Stress cardiograms have become the darlings of a fit-conscious world. Many corporations require them, and many people run out to get one the minute they turn 35 or 40. While they are *not* necessary for everyone, they can mean the difference between life and death when they're used appropriately.

When Should You Consider Taking a Stress Cardiogram?

1. If you have symptoms that could be due to heart disease, such as chest pain or shortness of breath, but your doctor hasn't been able to diagnose their cause with other noninvasive tests, such as a resting or ambulatory cardiogram.

2. If you are over 40 and among those people considered to be at "high risk" for heart disease because you have at least *two* of the following risk factors:
   - A family history of heart problems—in close family members under the age of 55
   - High cholesterol
   - High blood pressure (over 160/90)
   - Diabetes or
   - Heavy tobacco use

   NOTE: some groups suggest that the test be done on high-risk people after the age of 35, but these groups are in the minority.

3. If you are known to have heart disease, but your treatment, progress and status need to be evaluated. Stress cardiograms under these circumstances may be dangerous but necessary. The decision should be made by an expert, your doctor or a cardiologist. You may need the test in the following circumstances:
   - A short time (three days to three weeks) after a heart attack, to determine whether you're in danger of having another attack or of developing complications such as heart rhythm abnormalities
   - Months after a heart attack, to evaluate your progress and treatment
   - Months and/or years after coronary bypass surgery, to evaluate the effects of treatment and your progress
   - Months and/or years after coronary angiography shows a blockage in a coronary artery, when medical rather than surgical treatment was chosen, to evaluate the treatment's progress

4. If you're over 40 and work as a pilot; policeman; fireman; bus, truck, or train driver; or any other occupation where your having a sudden heart attack could endanger others.

5. If you're over 40, have not exerted yourself for a long period of time, have at least *one* risk factor (including diabetes, high blood pressure, tobacco use, high cholesterol, a family history of heart problems) and plan to begin a program of vigorous physical exercise. Some experts suggest that a stress cardiogram should be done at age 40 if you plan to start exercising, even if you don't have any risk factors.

Discuss your individual situation and the advantages and disadvantages of doing the test with your doctor.

When Not to Have a Stress Cardiogram

1. If you have unstable heart disease, congestive heart failure, significant abnormal heart rhythms, or diseases of the heart valves, unless you have been cleared to have the test by a cardiologist.

2. If you can't exercise, because of physical incapacity such as arthritis, amputation, peripheral vascular disease, or lung disease. In many of these cases, if the test is deemed necessary, medication can be used to stress the heart instead of exercise. Such medication can't be used if you're using the asthma drug theophylline.
3. If you're a healthy 35-year-old person with no symptoms or physical findings of heart disease, no major risk factors and no family or personal history of heart problems. In these circumstances, false positives are a real possibility, and most experts believe that the test is not worth the heartache, the cost, and the danger.
4. If you're a young, healthy woman without risk factors. Before menopause, women are less likely than men to have silent heart problems, and stress cardiograms on them are more likely to produce false positives. If you do have symptoms or risk factors, or if you're excessively concerned as you reach 40, discuss the test with your doctor.

What to Do If You're Told That Your Stress Test Is Positive

1. Keep in mind the percentage of false positives and discuss this likelihood with your doctor.
2. If you have no symptoms and no risk factors, do not act rashly. Remember there is a 10 to 25 percent chance that the test is wrong.
3. If you do decide to proceed, discuss the possibility of a treadmill thallium or thallium-SPECT test (discussed later in this chapter) with your doctor. When these tests are used in conjunction with the stress cardiogram, the overall accuracy is improved.

QUANTITATIVE TREADMILL TESTS

This is a new test using scoring and computer analysis to improve the accuracy of the standard stress test. It is performed in exactly the same way as the stress cardiogram, but it is interpreted differently. Some reports state that the quantitative tests resulted in fewer than 1 percent false positives, but others suggest that the test does not improve accuracy in patients who have no prior history of heart disease.

CARDIAC IMAGING

Between the "noninvasive" tests such as resting and exercise electrocardiograms (which are relatively safe but somewhat inaccurate) and the accurate but slightly dangerous procedures such as coronary angiography (see page 113) lies the whole new world of "cardiac imaging."

Cardiac imaging tests, which are already being used in conjunction with the older procedures, improve our ability to detect and treat heart disease by producing clearer, more precise views of our heart than could ever be accomplished with simple x-rays. (See page 159 for a more detailed explanation of the nature of imaging.)

THALLIUM TESTS (COLD-SPOT IMAGING)

Thallium is a radioactive element that accumulates in normal heart muscle, but not in heart muscle that has been injured by a heart attack or is endangered by decreased blood supply. This fact has allowed thallium testing to develop into a crucial diagnostic heart test over the past ten years.

What Is the Purpose of the Test?

Thallium scans are performed to detect "dead" heart muscle or heart muscle that does not receive enough blood. Since thallium will not collect in these areas, they will look "cold" on the scan, hence the term "cold-spot imaging." Resting thallium tests will show areas that are getting too little blood while the heart is resting. Exercise thallium tests are used to detect "cold" or endangered areas that don't show on "resting" thallium tests, in much the same way that stress cardiograms may discover changes not detected by resting cardiograms. "Redistribution" scans are used to distinguish between endangered and dead areas. If an area that was "cold" when you experienced symptoms or exercised becomes "hot" (fills with thallium) when you rest or the symptoms subside, it probably means that the area is endangered by a reduced blood supply when you exercise. If it stays cold, that part of the muscle has either died or is receiving no blood supply at all. This determination is invaluable when planning further tests and treatment.

How Is the Test Performed?

You will probably be instructed not to eat for a few hours before the test. For a "resting" thallium test, the doctor will inject a small amount of thallium into one of your veins while you are at rest. A special monitor will record the thallium's activity as it makes its way to and through your heart.

If an "exercise" thallium test is required, you will be asked to exercise, much as you did for the stress cardiogram, and the thallium will be injected after you reach maximum exercise tolerance or when you develop symptoms. The special monitor will scan the thallium's activity, as it did during the resting test.

A "redistribution" scan might be taken about three hours later and repeated the next day to aid in the accuracy and specificity of diagnosis.

If a delayed "redistribution" test is ordered, you will certainly be instructed to abstain from eating carbohydrates between tests, since they can interfere with the test's accuracy.

Where and by Whom Should the Test Be Performed and Interpreted?

Thallium testing is usually performed in a hospital, since it involves the use of an expensive monitor and the thallium is radioactive. The test may take half a day or even a whole day to perform, but you shouldn't have to stay in the hospital overnight. Like a stress cardiogram, this test should be performed by a properly trained technician, with a doctor present, and the results should be interpreted by an expert—a nuclear cardiologist or radiologist who specializes in this type of test.

How Accurate Is the Test?

When thallium testing is done alone, it's as accurate or slightly more accurate than stress cardiograms. When it's used to confirm or clarify a diagnosis after a stress cardiogram, it's far more accurate. Most studies report less than 10 percent "false positives" in patients who don't have symptoms and even fewer in those who do. Thallium testing does have its limitations, however. It is more expensive and more difficult to do than stress cardiograms. Also, it's not quite as accurate in women as it is in men, or in people with certain types of congestive heart failure or heart-valve diseases.

It is possible, although unlikely, for subtle heart disease to remain undetected even after thallium testing.

What Are the Dangers of Doing the Test?

The resting and redistribution thallium scans are very safe. The risks to your heart during exercise thallium testing are roughly the same as those during a stress cardiogram. The danger of heart attack and death is about .01 percent.

Is It Really Necessary?

Thallium heart testing is not routine, but it is useful for solving a wide variety of diagnostic dilemmas, and many experts consider it appropriate in the following circumstances:

1. To clarify the results or make a more precise diagnosis after a positive stress cardiogram in patients who do not have symptoms. Thallium can help to determine whether disease is really present and provide more information about its extent and location and whether or not it's reversible.
2. To clarify unclear findings of a coronary angiography (see page 113). If coronary angiography revealed a blockage, but your doctor was unsure whether or not the blockage was actually endangering a part of your heart, a thallium scan might answer the question for him.
3. To evaluate the cause and extent of disease in patients with known heart problems. Thallium would be used in these patients only when symptoms, a cardiogram, or simple exercise tests didn't lead to diagnosis and treatment.
4. To follow progress and treatment during medical treatment, or after balloon angioplasty or bypass surgery.
5. After a heart attack, to determine the risk of complications. The resting thallium scan can give more information than a resting cardiogram, and both are less dangerous than an exercise cardiogram in the period immediately following a heart attack.

Rarely, resting thallium scans may also be used to diagnose acute heart attacks in cases where all other tests are equivocal. Most experts feel that technetium imaging (see page 105) is better for that purpose in the first week after a suspected heart attack, while thallium is superior later on.

THALLIUM-SPECT IMAGING

While thallium testing may tell your doctor whether or not you have coronary artery disease, and whether or not it's reversible, a new test, called thallium-SPECT may do far more. SPECT stands for Single Photon Emission Computerized Transaxial Tomography. The test, which begins with an injection of thallium, uses a special tomographic x-ray machine (see page 173 for a detailed explanation of how tomography works) to monitor the accumulation of the substance within the heart.

This combination produces numerous views of the *inside* of the heart that provide information not only about whether a problem exists, but precisely where it begins and where it ends.

Thallium-SPECT is proving more accurate than resting thallium tests, but it is more expensive and more difficult to perform. It may be used more frequently in the near future.

RESTING TECHNETIUM SCAN

Like thallium, technetium is a radioactive tracer element that can be used to clarify the diagnosis of heart-related problems. Unlike thallium, technetium is absorbed by the *dead* cells—so that technetium scanning shows "hot" areas where there's a problem, rather than "cold."

What Is the Purpose of the Test?

Because technetium collects in diseased or dead heart cells, it may be used to confirm a heart attack if cardiograms or blood tests have been unable to make the diagnosis. The test must take place during a "window" of time from about two days to one week after the event, since that is the only time it will read positive. It may also be used when the cardiogram is *unreliable* for the diagnosis of heart attacks, such as when certain abnormalities in the heart's electrical conduction occur.

How Is the Test Performed?

Technetium is injected into one of your veins, and you are asked to lie still as a special monitor scans the accumulation of the substance within your heart. You may be asked not to eat immediately before the exam, but you don't have to avoid specific foods as you would for a thallium test.

Where and by Whom Should the Test Be Performed and Interpreted?

As with a thallium scan, this procedure is usually performed in a hospital. It is administered by a technician, and should be interpreted by an expert—a nuclear cardiologist or radiologist who specializes in this test.

How Accurate Is the Test?

A technetium scan produces 15 to 20 percent false positive results and about 10 percent false negatives. The results must be confirmed with history, cardiogram and other tests.

What Are the Dangers of Doing the Test?

The dangers here are minor: the radiation dose is small (about the same as for a chest x-ray), and there is a minor possibility of an allergic reaction.

Is It Really Necessary?

The resting technetium scan may be necessary to diagnose heart attacks only when the less expensive tests, such as heart enzymes (page 208) and resting cardiograms, do not produce a definite diagnosis.

On rare occasions, it is used sometime after a heart attack to evaluate persistent problems; also, when used in conjunction with wall-motion studies (see following section), it may provide valuable information.

MULTIPLE-GATED HEART SCAN (MUGA)

This test uses the patient's own blood cells, after they've been radioactively labeled, to examine the heart's performance.

What Is the Purpose of the Test?

The MUGA test is unique. While exercise testing may determine whether there is decreased blood flow, and thallium can determine whether the decrease is reversible, the MUGA can watch your heart in action.

It can study heart-wall motion that could indicate damage or decreased blood flow to the wall and it may be utilized to diagnose blockage in the coronary arteries. It can compute your "ejection fraction," a measure of how much blood your heart pumps with each beat. This is invaluable information that helps doctors to determine the strength of your heart and whether or not you have any heart failure.

How Is the Test Performed?

Your doctor or a technician will take a sample of your blood, which he will then expose to a minute amount of radiation, usually by adding radioactive technetium. This blood is then injected back into a vein and studied by multiple scans as it moves through your heart. An electrocardiogram is run simultaneously, and it is used to trigger the scans and study the heart while it works. A computer sums up the scans and "gates" them, i.e., correlates them with parts of your heart cycle.

Where and by Whom Should the Test Be Done and Interpreted?

The test may be administered by a technician, usually in a hospital, but it should be interpreted by an expert: a nuclear cardiologist or a radiologist who specializes in this type of test.

How Accurate Is the Test?

MUGA scans are highly accurate in the detection of wall-motion abnormalities and the determination of ejection fraction.

What Are the Dangers of Doing the Test?

The risks of a MUGA scan are minor; they encompass the rare possibility of infection or bleeding at the injection site and radiation exposure roughly equal to that of a chest x-ray.

Is It Really Necessary?

The MUGA is not a routine test for use on patients without known or suspected heart disease, but in patients at risk for heart disease, it can provide information that cannot be duplicated by other types of tests and is appropriate in the following circumstances.

1. To evaluate heart performance.
   - To compute ejection fraction and determine if heart failure exists
   - To evaluate heart size and motion
   - To assess the function of the heart when other tests have discovered an abnormality, such as a partial blockage found during thallium testing or angiography
   - To follow a patient's progress and the results of medical or surgical treatment
2. To determine whether an aneurysm exists; an aneurysm is a dangerous weakness in the heart wall that may occur spontaneously or after a heart attack.
3. As an adjunct in the diagnosis of heart attack when other tests have not made an unequivocal diagnosis.

ECHOCARDIOGRAMS (ULTRASOUND TESTS)

You may have seen movies about submarines or read the book *Hunt for Red October* by Tom Clancy, in which the submarine commanders bounced sound waves off the hulls of enemy ships in order to locate them by the echo produced. The echocardiogram operates on the same principle, bouncing ultra-high-frequency sound waves against the heart and then forming an image from the echos that return.

Echocardiograms, which are a type of ultrasound test (see page 172), are the most commonly used noninvasive cardiac imaging test in use today. They are very valuable for the detection of a number of different heart abnormalities, and may be risk-free.

What Is the Purpose of the Test?

Two types of sound-wave imagings are currently in use. The m-mode produces flat images of the heart; the more recently developed "2d"— for two-dimensional— allows the doctor to watch the heart in action and record its movements. The resulting sound pictures can be used to evaluate suspected valve disease, and to investigate murmurs, clicks, and unexplained chest pains.

With them, a doctor can study the size of the heart's various chambers and determine whether an infection is present on one of the valves, or if there is excessive fluid around the heart.

Both tests can also be employed to search for heart tumors and recently they have been used along with other tests to evaluate the possibility of coronary artery disease.

How Is the Test Performed?

The echocardiogram is performed as you lie on a bed or table, hooked up to an electrocardiogram via electrodes taped to your arms and legs. The doctor or technician presses a small machine called a "transducer" against your chest, then moves it around in the area of your heart, sending out soundwaves, picking up the echos, and transmitting the results to a monitor screen.

The difference between the "m-mode" and the "second-dimensional" echocardiograms is in the type of machine and monitor used; you will not experience any difference during the performance of the test.

Where and by Whom Should the Test Be Performed and Interpreted?

An echocardiogram can be administered by a qualified technician in a hospital or clinic, and you don't need to stay overnight. It must be interpreted by a doctor who is trained in the interpretation of echocardiograms.

How Accurate Is the Test?

The accuracy of echocardiograms is limited in 10 to 20 percent of patients:

- Those who are extremely overweight
- Those who have had chest surgery
- Those who have a history of chronic lung problems

These problems do not affect the accuracy of other imaging procedures as much.

In other people, echocardiograms are considered very accurate for the evaluation of heart-valve problems and abnormalities of wall motion. Their accuracy in the detection of coronary artery disease depends on the detection of heart-wall motion abnormalities, and they have been found to be as reliable as the MUGA scan for that purpose.

What Are the Dangers of Doing the Test?

Most scientists consider echocardiograms virtually risk-free. Some have raised questions about the long-term use of sound waves, but no adverse effects have been proven and the most in-depth studies have so far cited only a "theoretical" danger.

Is It Really Necessary?

The echocardiogram is not a routine test, but it has definite uses. It may be appropriate in the following situations:

1. In anyone suspected of having valvular disease, including anyone with symptoms of mitral valve prolapse, such as palpitations, unexplained losses of consciousness, fast heart beat, or unexplained nausea, vomiting, and chest pain.
2. In the diagnosis of "endocarditis," an infection of the heart valves. In this case, bacterial growths on the valves can actually be seen with the echocardiogram, although confirming blood cultures are necessary as well.
3. Evaluation of the inner wall of your heart (its septum) for holes, growths, or thickening.
4. Evaluation of the cause of unexplained chest pain when other, less expensive tests such as resting or exercise cardiograms have been unable to produce a diagnosis.
5. Evaluation of congenital heart disease or complications of heart attack such as aneurysms.

Note that in the case of both Number 4 and Number 5, MUGA scans may be more accurate for the obese patient or one who has chronic lung disease or a history of chest surgery.

DOPPLER AND COLOR-FLOW MAPPING OF THE HEART

These new tests use a digital scanner to turn the echos that are received from the heart during ultrasound studies into a precise (and sometimes multicolored) picture that provides specific information about the heart's blood flow. Because they involve no risk, the tests may be preferable to the more dangerous catheterization studies for certain individuals, such as infants or adults who are seriously ill from heart disease. Doppler and Color-flow mapping are now being used to study problems of the pericardium, the tissue that lines the outside of the heart, and to provide crucial information about the flow of blood across diseased heart valves. Most experts feel that both tests will also become valuable tools in the detection and evaluation of congenital heart problems and diseases of the aorta, the largest artery in your body.

ELECTROPHYSIOLOGICAL (EPS) TESTING OR MAPPING

Your heart pumps blood as a result of an electrical impulse that is generated from the top of the heart and moves down and around your heart muscle, causing it to contract. The wavy lines you see on an electrocardiogram are the machine's interpretation of this electrical impulse. While an electrocardiogram allows a doctor to detect cells that are endangered by a decrease in blood flow, electrophysiological testing allows him to make a specific study of the electrical pathway itself.

What Is the Purpose of the Test?

EPS is used to evaluate disorders of rhythm that do not respond to conventional treatment. It may also be used in the diagnosis of certain complex disorders of conduction, including a condition called Wolff Parkinson White syndrome, which can result in disorders of the heart's rhythm.

How Is the Test Performed?

You'll lie on a bed while a doctor inserts a microfine wire into a blood vessel into your arm or groin, then painlessly guides it into your heart by using an x-ray monitor. With the wire in place, controlled electrical pulses will be used to stimulate your heart, and its electrical conduction system will be studied and mapped.

Where and by Whom Should the Test Be Performed and Interpreted?

This test should be done in a hospital by a cardiologist who is specially trained in EPS.

How Accurate Is the Test?

EPS is the most specific, accurate method for studying the electrical pathway of your heart.

What Are the Dangers of Doing the Test?

EPS can be dangerous. It can cause heart arrhythmias, heart attack, and even death. These risks are all significantly less when the EPS is performed by an expert who has extensive experience with the procedure.

Is It Really Necessary?

This test should be reserved for intractable, unresponsive, or repetitive problems of heart rhythm where other diagnostic methods have failed to provide enough information.

NEWER IMAGING TESTS FOR THE HEART

PET (Positron Emission Tomography) Scan of the Heart

PET scans use radioactively labeled biological substances, such as sugar, to study the actual metabolic activity of organs. During a heart PET scan, you will receive an injection of such a substance, and special tomographic monitors will detect the radiation as it passes through your heart. These monitors will produce special x-ray pictures of your heart in which shadows of structures in front of and behind the section under scrutiny do not show. (For a complete discussion of tomography, see page 173.)

The scans are expensive: there are currently only seventeen PET scanners in the United States. But because they may provide early, subtle information about the heart's function, experts feel that PET scans will become a valuable tool in the diagnosis and treatment of heart disease, and many more are being built. For a more detailed description of PET scans and their use in studying other internal organs, see page 180.

CINE CT (Computerized Tomography) of the Heart

This test, also called "ultrafast computed tomography," combines a computerized axial tomography, or CAT scanner, with an electron beam to study the structure, function, and blood flow in and to the heart. As with a "dye-enhanced" CAT scan (see page 175), you're given an injection, then lie still on a table as the machine takes multiple x-rays of your heart. The radiation exposure is about the same as with a regular CAT scan of the chest.

The Cine CT has been used to examine the coronary arteries of patients after bypass surgery, to determine whether any new blockages have developed to study the heart's valves and walls, and to determine whether there's any disease of the pericardium, the tissue that lines the outside of the heart. Cine CT is still in its infancy, but experts feel that it will be used on a regular basis in the not-too-distant future.

MAGNETIC RESONANCE IMAGING (MRI) OF THE HEART

Magnetic Resonance Imaging enables doctors to view internal organs in a completely different way than other noninvasive tests. Through the use of electrical waves and a giant magnetic field, MRI machines cause the protons of your internal organs to move and emit energy that can be detected and analyzed on a large computer screen.

This test doesn't require painful injections and it doesn't expose you to dangerous radiation, but an MRI cannot be performed on people with heart pacemakers, metal-containing IUD's, or metal clips on blood vessels from previous surgery, since the magnet can affect these devices adversely.

MRI has already become established as a major diagnostic tool in the evaluation of the brain and bone abnormalities, but it's just beginning to be used for the detection of heart disease. Once it has been established and studied, experts feel that it will add a highly precise, virtually risk-free tool to cardiac diagnosis.

For a full description of MRI and its use in other parts of the body, see page 177.

ANGIOGRAPHY

Angiography is the study of blood vessels through the injection of a dye that can be seen on an x-ray.

Coronary Angiography

Coronary angiography involves injecting a dye into the coronary arteries, to determine whether they're blocked, whether your heart muscle and life are endangered. It can also be used to study the passage of blood through the heart, and the performance of the heart as it beats.

What Is the Purpose of the Test?

Coronary angiography is the definitive test for the study of coronary artery blood flow. It determines whether there is a blockage, how bad the blockage is, how many and which arteries are blocked, and whether medications or surgery are needed. Cardiac catheterization, the portion of the test where the dye passes into your heart, can be used to study the walls and chambers of the heart as it beats.

How Is the Test Performed?

First, you're connected to an electrocardiogram, then a doctor or technician inserts a small needle into your vein so you can be given medications or fluids in the course of the test.

Next, you're given local numbing medicine (most patients are awake for the procedure), an incision is made, and a larger needle is inserted into a blood vessel in your arm or groin. A tube (catheter) and microfine wire are passed into the opening and threaded to your coronary arteries using x-ray guidance.

Then the doctor injects the dye—you may feel a warm "flush" in your chest and head, but usually no pain—and moving x-ray films are taken as it passes through your arteries. The injection may be repeated several times, and films will also be taken as the dye moves through your heart. These films are then carefully studied by a team of experts.

Where and by Whom Should the Test Be Performed and Interpreted?

Coronary angiography must be done in the special catheterization lab of a hospital.

It should be performed and interpreted by a specialist—a radiologist or specially trained cardiologist.

How Accurate Is the Test?

Very.

Coronary angiography allows the doctor to see virtually 100 percent of blockages. Although the exact extent of the blockage is sometimes difficult to determine, angiography can usually provide enough information to tell the doctor whether you're in the danger zone.

The cardiac catheterization portion of the test is accurate for the study of heart-wall motion and flow abnormalities that might occur in valvular disease or when tiny holes exist in the heart walls.

What Are the Dangers of Doing the Test?

The danger of a "major complication" during coronary angiography, such as blood clot, allergic reaction, stroke, heart attack, perforation, or heart injury or infection is small but real. However, the extent of these dangers depends on the experience of the person performing the test. Risk is lowest in testing centers that have the most experience with the procedure.

The dangers are greatest among high-risk people: those over the age of 60, with severe coronary disease, or congestive heart failure.

Is It Really Necessary?

Since it is currently the most definitive test for coronary artery disease, coronary angiography is necessary for certain people.

However, some studies have shown that it is used inappropriately nearly 17 percent of the time. Others have reported that it is negative 12 to 37 percent of the time when it's done on people who have no symptoms. For these reasons, and because of the test's inherent risks, it is imperative that it only be performed under two circumstances:

● To evaluate chest pain and coronary artery blockage when other tests have not produced a precise, definitive diagnosis
● When the results of the angiogram might affect treatment decisions

In other words, no matter how high the likelihood of disease, and no matter how bad the problem is, angiography should not be done if the doctors tell you that your medical or surgical treatment will be the same, no matter what the test shows.

OTHER FORMS OF ANGIOGRAPHY

Carotid Angiography

This test, which studies the blood vessels in your neck that bring blood to the brain, is done when your doctor suspects that a blockage in one of the vessels has caused, or may place you in danger of, a stroke.

Cerebral Angiography

Cerebral angiography is used to study the blood vessels within the brain in order to evaluate the size or exact location of a tumor, to search for the source of a hemorrhage, or to detect aneurysms—weaknesses in brain blood vessels that are liable to burst and cause hemorrhage.

Aortography

Aortography is used to study the largest artery in your body, the aorta, for signs of injury, disease, widening, or weakness.

Angiographies can also be done on the abdomen or arms and legs as well as the blood vessels of many internal organs, such as the kidney, lungs, or intestines.

Digital Subtraction Angiography (DSA)—The Newest Form of Angiography

Angiography is a highly specific, highly accurate test, but it has its limitations. Unwanted shadows and bone may obscure the x-ray image, making it hard to interpret. Digital subtraction angiography solves that problem by using a combination of television and high-speed digital computer technology to subtract the unwanted images and produce a clearer, more precise, image.

What Is the Purpose of the Test?

DSA is used for the same purposes as all other angiographies, to determine whether there is a blockage in a blood vessel, to visualize a weakness such as an aneurysm, an abnormality, or a tumor. It can be used for evaluating the coronary arteries, the heart, the kidneys, and other internal organs.

How Is the Test Performed?

As you lie in bed, intravenous injections of dye are made into two different blood vessels. The dye is more diluted than with regular angiography, but repeated, larger amounts, or "bolus" injections, may be necessary for some studies. You lie still while the computer and x-ray machine evaluates the images and subtracts unwanted shadows. The picture thus displays more of the blood vessels and less of the surrounding tissue.

How Accurate Is the Test?

DSA is a new procedure, and its accuracy has not been subjected to extensive studies. However, most experts feel it will turn out to be at least as accurate as regular angiography.

What Are the Dangers of the Test?

The dangers are similar to those of regular angiography: infection or bleeding at the injection site, perforation of a blood vessel, allergic reaction, or clot formation. If bolus injections are used, there may be an added danger of fluid or contrast overload, which could affect your heart or kidneys. As with regular angiographies, you can minimize the risks by making sure that an expert performs the test.

Is It Really Necessary?

DSA is not presently a first line test. However, in the future it may be used to study the blood vessels when less complex or dangerous tests cannot produce a diagnosis.

THE MOST IMPORTANT HEART TESTS FOR YOUR QUICK REFERENCE

- The *resting electrocardiogram* provides direct information about your heart's rate, rhythm, and electrical activity while you rest. It can also provide indirect information about blood flow, the health of the heart muscle, and areas of muscle death.
- The *ambulatory electrocardiogram* monitors the same information over the course of an entire day, and correlates changes with your activity or the occurrence of specific symptoms.
- A *stress electrocardiogram* provides the same type of information about your heart while you exercise.
- The *thallium test* provides specific information about the blood flow to

an area, and whether the muscle in that area is already dead or just endangered.

- The *resting technetium scan* tells us if an area of the muscle is diseased or has died.
- The *MUGA test* shows us the blood inside the heart, and tells us about heart failure, muscle strength, and wall motion.
- The *echocardiogram* provides information about your heart valves, the inner wall of your heart, and wall motion. It may also be used along with other tests to evaluate the possibility of coronary artery disease.
- The *Thallium-SPECT* test uses a special tomographic machine to provide more precise information than is gathered by a resting thallium test.

EIGHT

Tests for Women

Medical science has made major progress in the prevention and cure of the diseases that are unique to women. Tests for a healthy baby and prospective mother during pregnancy, and for the early detection of cancer in women are among our safest and most accurate screening tests. Even so, in no area is there more need for improvement.

One out of every ten women in the United States will get breast cancer during her lifetime. One hundred and twenty thousand new cases will be diagnosed this year alone, and more than 40,000 will be fatal; but the American Cancer Society (ACS) estimates that a large percentage of those women could be saved by early detection and treatment. The death rate from cancer of the cervix has decreased by 70 percent in the past 40 years, mainly because of the routine use of the simple, safe Pap smear, yet nearly one out of five American women do not get regular Pap smears. New tests for the early, safe diagnosis of fetal abnormalities and potential dangers during pregnancy have been approved, yet studies show that many women have no idea which tests to choose. If you learn which of the tests that evaluate problems unique to women are necessary for you and when they should be done, you'll decrease your chances of developing a serious illness, and increase your chances of recovering, should one occur.

THE PAP SMEAR

The Pap smear is a safe, simple test for the early detection of cervical cancer. Since it was first introduced in 1948 by Dr. George Papanicolaou, nearly 400 million have been done. But recent reports of laboratory errors have cast a shadow over its previously untarnished image, and many women still do not understand the suggested guidelines for its use and interpretation.

What Is the Purpose of the Test?

The purpose of the Pap smear is to provide early detection of cervical cancer—while it is still curable. It may also be used to detect cervical inflammation or infection, and to evaluate how the cervix is responding to certain treatments.

How Is the Test Performed?

The Pap smear is taken during a pelvic exam. You will be asked to lie on your back on the examining table, with your feet supported in stirrups. A small instrument called a speculum will be used to hold your vagina open while a cotton swab or spatula is used to take cell samples from the cervix. These samples will then be sent to a special laboratory for examination. The results are usually returned within a week to ten days.

Where and by Whom Should the Test Be Performed and Interpreted?

The Pap smear should be taken in the doctor's office by a gynecologist, private or family doctor, or by a nurse practitioner. This is a test calling for delicacy and sensitivity on the part of the person who administers it, and you should choose someone you can trust and with whom you feel comfortable.

The samples should be examined and evaluated in the lab by a doctor who is a specialist in pathology, or by a trained technician.

How Accurate Is the Test?

Studies have shown that you can assure the accuracy of your Pap smear by taking the following steps:

1. Make sure your doctor is well acquainted with the laboratory where he sends the samples, and knows their reputation.
2. Ask whether the laboratory has adequate numbers of technicians to handle the volume of tests they study. Research has shown that overworked technicians make more mistakes.
3. Ask whether the lab is licensed and whether it has ever been inspected.

4. Ask him whether the laboratory routinely "rescreens" negative tests and whether they perform regular reexaminations on abnormal results. These practices drive the danger of error down even further.
5. If you have any doubts about the results, ask that the test be sent to another laboratory for confirmation.

What Are the Dangers of Doing the Test?

The test may cause slight discomfort, and a little bleeding afterward, but it is basically very safe, and there is no evidence of any long-term ill effects.

Is It Really Necessary?

According to the American Cancer Society (ACS), women who are sexually active or have reached the age of 18 should have an annual Pap smear and pelvic exam.

After three consecutive normal exams, the tests may be performed less frequently. The American College of Obstetricians and Gynecologists (ACOG) recommends more frequent testing—once a year after the age of 18. Both organizations recommend yearly pelvic exams after the age of 40. Although many women who pass menopause or have hysterectomies choose to cease getting Pap smears, recent evidence suggests that they too may require occasional testing to screen for vaginal cancer. The ACS and ACOG are careful to point out that this schedule should be modified according to individual history and risk.

If you are in any of the following high-risk groups, Pap smears may have to be performed sooner, and more frequently.

- Women who have multiple sex partners (including women under the age of 18)
- Women who first had sexual intercourse at an early age
- Women who have a personal history of cervical or uterine cancer, genital herpes, or warts
- Women whose mothers took Diethylstilbestrol (DES) during pregnancy
- Any woman who has ever had an abnormal Pap smear result

What You Should Know and Do About Pap Smear Results

Approximately ninety percent of Pap smear results are read as normal: no cancerous or atypical cells are found. Five to six percent reveal "inflammatory" cells—cells which show some microscopic changes but are not cancerous. Three to four percent indicate the presence of what are known as "precancerous" cells, and about .1 percent (one out of 1,000 tests) show the presence of malignancies.

Laboratories usually report the results in one of the following ways:

- Normal.
- Atypical cells, no cancerous cells present.
- Cercival intraepithelial neoplasia; these refer to precancerous lesions. This class may be subdivided into further descriptive categories, depending on how deep the changes go.
- Carcinoma in situ; localized cancer.
- Invasive cancer.

You should not be unduly alarmed by abnormal results; the Pap smear is meant as a screening test only. The false negative rate (abnormal cells that are missed) for "normal" readings is small, but the "false positive" rate may be higher for the other classes.

The majority of women with abnormal Pap smears do not turn out to have serious cancer.

You can sift through the confusion, and make sure that your Pap smear results in proper action, by observing the following simple guidelines.

IF YOUR PAP SMEAR IS READ AS NORMAL
1. Continue to follow the guidelines for routine Pap smears, and your doctor's recommendations.
2. If you develop symptoms such as pelvic pain, discharge, or bleeding, discuss the need for a repeat exam, no matter what your previous results were.

IF YOUR PAP SMEAR IS READ AS ABNORMAL
1. Take the steps listed above which are considered necessary to ensure the accuracy of your reporting laboratory.
2. Have the test repeated.
3. If, on repeat testing, your Pap smear is abnormal, discuss the need for further tests with your doctor.

Do not proceed to surgery until such confirming tests are run.

COLPOSCOPY

Colposcopy is a simple, safe procedure that many doctors use along with Pap smears to aid in the early detection of cervical cancer.

What Is the Purpose of the Test?

Colposcopy is used in the United States mainly to confirm the results of abnormal Pap smears and to determine the extent of abnormality. More recently, it has been used to identify venereal warts *(Condylomata accuminata)*, which are associated with an increased risk of cervical cancer.

How Is the Test Performed?

The test is done during a pelvic exam. A diluted solution of vinegar is gently applied to the area being tested (the external genitalia or the cervix) to remove mucus and facilitate examination. The culposcope, a magnifying scope with a special light attached, is then used to examine the area and determine whether there are any areas of abnormality not visible to the naked eye.

Where and by Whom Should the Test Be Performed and Interpreted?

For women, your primary-care physician or gynecologist can perform the colposcopy, but its use and interpretation take a high level of expertise. Make sure he has studied this particular procedure before having it performed.

How Accurate Is the Test?

When done correctly, colposcopy is as accurate as a Pap smear, but it requires a higher level of expertise to perform. When used to confirm a Pap smear, it can increase overall accuracy in the early detection of cancers. Many experts feel that it is accurate for the diagnosis of venereal warts as well, but so far there have been no controlled studies that evaluate its effectiveness in this area.

What Are the Dangers of Doing the Test?

Occasional irritation and allergic reactions to the acetic acid have been reported. If biopsies are done when an abnormal area is identified, there may be some bleeding and risk of infection, but no long-term adverse effects have been associated with colposcopies.

Is It Really Necessary?

Only in certain cases. Colposcopy is performed routinely in Europe, but experts in the United States do not believe that its value warrants its cost as a routine screening procedure. It costs approximately fifteen times as much as a Pap smear, and when used alone as screening test, it has not proved to be more accurate. As an adjunct, after an abnormal Pap smear, or in those cases where the diagnosis is in question, colposcopy may prove invaluable.

Since many scientists believe that venereal warts may be associated with an increased risk of cervical cancer, and these warts are invisible to the human eye in 25 percent of cases, colposcopy may be indicated in people who have a history of venereal warts or have been exposed to them during sexual activity.

ENDOMETRIAL TISSUE SAMPLE

Endometrial tissue lines the inside of the uterus. It contracts, changes, and bleeds in response to both normal and abnormal stimulation by the body's hormones.

What Is the Purpose of the Test?

Endometrial tissue sampling is done for a number of reasons.

1. To diagnose (and occasionally to treat) the cause of abnormal uterine bleeding.
2. To screen for cancer of the uterus in postmenopausal women.
3. To aid in the diagnosis of infertility. In this case, the test is used to determine whether the endometrium is in sync with the rest of the woman's menstrual cycle and able to accept the implantation of an embryo.

How Is the Test Performed?

The sample is taken during a pelvic examination. The doctor passes a thin tube through your cervix into your uterus and gently vacuums out a thin layer of endometrial tissue. You may feel mild to moderate cramping during the procedure. If the test is done during a dilatation and curettage (D&C), progressively larger instruments will be used to dilate, or enlarge, your cervix, and the endometrial layer will be scraped rather than suctioned. Hysteroscopy (see page 147) and endometrial laser ablation are newer procedures that may either replace D&C or be used along with it. In these cases, an instrument is used to view the uterine lining while treating it for abnormal bleeding or other gynecological problems.

Where and by Whom Should the Test Be Performed and Interpreted?

The test may be performed in your doctor's office, a hospital, or in a clinic. It should be done and interpreted by a doctor who is experienced with the procedure.

How Accurate Is the Test?

The endometrial tissue sample is accurate for the diagnosis of cancer—when a good sample is obtained. If, however, the test is done blind (without viewing through a scope), or if an inadequate sample is obtained during suction, the specific diagnosis may be missed. Accuracy can be enhanced with a viewing scope and by making sure that an expert performs and interprets the test.

What Are the Dangers of Doing the Test?

This test can sometimes result in prolonged bleeding afterward, and there's a small possibility of infection. Very rarely, the cervix is torn or the uterus perforated in the course of the procedure.

If performed during the early stages of pregnancy, it may result in a miscarriage. If there's any chance that you're pregnant, make sure that you have a pregnancy test before the sample is taken.

Is It Really Necessary?

Endometrial tissue sampling is not recommended on a routine basis. However, since abnormal uterine bleeding is one of the most common signs of cancer of the uterus, and because the disease can spread before it causes bleeding, the test may be recommended for the following women:

1. High-risk, postmenopausal women—as a screening test; whether or not bleeding is present
   ● Women who are extremely overweight
   ● Women with diabetes
   ● Women who have never been pregnant
   ● Women on hormone therapy

2. Premenopausal women, when other tests have failed to yield a diagnosis
   - To diagnose the cause of infertility
   - To diagnose and treat abnormal uterine bleeding

   In all of these cases, you should discuss the method for obtaining the sample with your doctor before having the test done. If simple suctioning is to be used, there's little danger. But if a D&C is to be performed, you may want to consider your options.

   In 1985, nearly 350,000 women underwent in-hospital diagnostic D&C for abnormal uterine bleeding, but many experts feel that the tissue sample is more safely and accurately obtained through hysteroscopy (see page 147).

MAMMOGRAM

Breast cancer is the second most common cancer in women, behind only lung cancer. Self-exam coupled with mammogram is the surest way to aid early diagnosis and increase your chances of cure.

What Is the Purpose of the Test?

The purpose of the test is the early detection of breast cancers—while they're still curable. Self-examination of the breast is crucial to early diagnosis, but because many curable breast cancers are smaller than 1 centimeter in diameter and may not be felt during self-examination, the mammogram is considered necessary by the American Cancer Society.

How Is the Test Performed?

You will be asked to undress, and each breast in turn will be pressed against an x-ray plate, using a special "compressor" to flatten out the tissue, while you hold your breath and an x-ray image is taken. You may find the compressor a little uncomfortable, and may feel minor pain.

Where and by Whom Should the Test Be Performed and Interpreted?

Mammograms can be done in a doctor's office, or in the x-ray department of a clinic or hospital.

An x-ray technician will perform the test, which should then be interpreted by an experienced doctor, usually a radiologist or surgeon.

How Accurate Is the Test?

Mammograms are highly accurate, but they may miss a small percentage of cancers. For that reason, they should be combined with regular self-examinations and examinations by your doctor. Also, you should ask for a repeat examination if you notice a lump, a change in your breasts, or any of the early warning signs, such as discharge, bleeding, or dimpling of the nipple.

What Are the Dangers of Doing the Test?

There is always some risk involved in any procedure that uses radiation; in this case the risk is simply not as great as the risk of having breast cancer and missing it.

Is It Really Necessary?

The ACS recommends that women have their first mammogram between the ages of 35 and 39, one every one to two years between the ages of 40 and 49, and one every year thereafter.

Women at high risk for breast cancer—those with a personal or family history of the disease—may require their first test sooner, and subsequent tests more frequently. This may also be advisable if you have large or lumpy breasts, not because they increase your risk, but simply because cancers may be more difficult for you or your doctor to feel during examination.

PELVIC ULTRASOUND

This procedure uses the same kind of sound waves as do other ultrasound tests (see page 172) to study the organs inside the pelvis—the bladder, uterus, the fallopian tubes, and the ovaries.

What Is the Purpose of the Test?

Pelvic ultrasounds are performed to diagnose difficult or subtle pelvic diseases such as tubal pregnancies, cysts, infections, and tumors.

They may also be used to determine whether you have a normal intrauterine pregnancy and to follow the course of certain high-risk pregnancies (see amniocentesis, page 129).

In addition, they may be used along with other tests to aid in the diagnosis of endometriosis.

How Is the Test Performed?

A transducer, much like a small tape recorder, is passed back and forth across your abdomen. This instrument bounces sound waves against the various organs and picks up their echos for transmission to a computer, which then translates them onto the screen of a special monitor.

In most cases, you will be asked to drink about five glasses of water an hour before the test so that your bladder will fill, allowing the radiologist to use it as a landmark on the test. In emergency situations, when there's no time to prepare, a catheter may be inserted through your uretha into the bladder to identify it instead.

The tube should be placed under sterile conditions by an expert, who will use special medicine to clean your urethra (the external opening to your bladder) before passing the tube in. If it's done properly, it should not result in undue pain, though it may cause you some discomfort.

Where and by Whom Should the Test Be Performed and Interpreted?

The test may be performed in a hospital, a doctor's office, or a clinic, by a specially trained ultrasound technician. The results should be interpreted by a radiologist, or a gynecologist who knows how to read ultrasound monitors.

How Accurate Is the Test?

Pelvic ultrasounds are extremely accurate for the detection of tumors, cysts, and both uterine and tubal pregnancies. They are less accurate for the diagnosis of infection and endometriosis, and should only be employed along with other tests for these purposes.

What Are the Dangers of Doing the Test?

Some scientists have theorized the possibility of long-term dangers to an unborn infant. To date, no controlled study has supported this theory, and there is no proof that ultrasound examinations endanger the woman on whom they are performed.

Is It Really Necessary?

Ultrasound examination may be necessary to investigate unexplained pain in the pelvic region, to rule out such possibilities as ectopic or tubal pregnancy, tumors, and infections, and to determine whether or not you are pregnant. Since it is considered safe, it should be used whenever these diagnoses are being considered and other, less expensive tests such as pelvic examination or blood and urine tests fail to make a diagnosis.

RUBELLA TESTING

German measles (also known as rubella) is not a major problem—unless you are pregnant. If you catch the disease then, it may cause irreversible damage to your unborn child.

What Is the Purpose of the Test?

The rubella test checks to see whether or not you have ever been exposed to rubella. If you have not, your doctor may recommend that you receive a vaccine before you get pregnant, to prevent you from catching it during pregnancy and to protect any future fetus.

How Is the Test Performed?

This simple test involves extracting a small quantity of blood from the arm. This blood is sent to a special laboratory to be tested for antibodies against the rubella virus; their presence is a sure sign that you have been exposed. The results are usually available within a week.

Where and by Whom Should the Test Be Performed and Interpreted?

A nurse or physician's assistant can take the sample in the doctor's office, a clinic, or a hospital. A blood technician in a laboratory will test it, and a pathologist or your family doctor will interpret the results.

How Accurate Is the Test?

The test is virtually 100 percent accurate for exposure to the virus. If you have antibodies, you don't need the vaccine.

What Are the Dangers of Doing the Test?

As with any blood test, the only dangers are slight pain during the test, and the possibility of local bleeding or infection if it's not performed properly.

Is It Really Necessary?

It may not be, if you know you've already had the German measles. However, since the danger involved in the test is slight in comparison with the risk you run by catching the German measles during pregnancy, it's wise to check anyway.

The rubella test needs to be performed only once—the antibodies last a lifetime. Have it done before you become pregnant, or early in pregnancy, if you become pregnant unexpectedly.

If you've never been exposed, the vaccine will not be administered while you're pregnant, but the knowledge of your vulnerability will ensure that you avoid anyone with the infection until your baby is born.

AMNIOCENTESIS

Since amniocentesis was developed more than thirty years ago, millions have been performed worldwide. It is a safe, accurate procedure for the detection of fetal health and may be used for certain types of treatment as well.

What Is the Purpose of the Test?

Amniocentesis is performed to evaluate the health of the growing baby and to diagnose genetic problems. It can provide evidence of such diverse problems as Down's syndrome, Tay-Sachs disease, and spina bifida.

In situations where the doctor is concerned about premature delivery, or if he believes that early delivery will be necessary, it can be used to determine whether or not the baby's lungs are developed enough to handle the outside world.

It may also be used for the diagnosis of womb infection, fetal distress late in pregnancy, or the determination of the baby's sex, if this is considered necessary for the baby's health. (See "Is It Really Necessary?" below.)

How Is the Test Performed?

Amniocentesis is generally performed after the sixteenth week of pregnancy. The doctor watches an ultrasound monitor as he guides a long, hollow needle into the amniotic sac that surrounds the baby. A small quantity of amniotic fluid is withdrawn for evaluation.

Where and by Whom Should the Test Be Performed and Interpreted?

The test may be done at a doctor's office, a clinic, or a hospital, but only by a physician who is specially trained in the performance of amniocentesis.

How Accurate Is the Test?

Amniocentesis is highly accurate for the diagnosis of fetal abnormalities. At present it is the most accurate method for the diagnosis of fetal maturity.

What Are the Dangers of Doing the Test?

When it was first developed, prospective mothers worried about the dangers to their unborn baby. Over the years, however, a less than 1 percent danger of miscarriage has been reported, and no other adverse effects on the baby have been discovered.

Is It Really Necessary?

Amniocentesis is most necessary to diagnose fetal distress, fetal infection, and fetal maturity when premature delivery is imminent. It is the procedure of choice when certain nervous system abnormalities, such as spina bifida, are suspected, since earlier fetal tests may not detect these problems (see chorionic villus sampling, below).

Also, amniocentesis is one of two procedures (see comparison of chorionic villus sampling and amniocentesis on page 132) that may be chosen to diagnose other genetic problems in high-risk pregnancies:

- When the mother is over age 35
- When there is a history of genetic defects in the mother and/or father's family
- When there is a history of many miscarriages

Amniocentesis is not routinely recommended solely for the determination of the baby's sex unless there is a history of a sex-linked disorder in the family.

CHORIONIC VILLUS SAMPLING (CVS)

Chorionic villus sampling is a new prenatal diagnostic procedure that may someday replace amniocentesis for the diagnosis of certain fetal problems. The chorion is an outer membrane of the embryo that plays a role in the formation of the placenta. "Villi" are the branchlike projections from the chorion into the placenta.

What Is the Purpose of the Test?

CVS can be used to diagnose many of the same abnormalities as amniocentesis. It cannot, however, be used to evaluate fetal maturity or spina bifida and other nervous system abnormalities.

How Is the Test Performed?

Unlike amniocentesis, CVS may be performed as early as the second month of pregnancy. A small, flexible tube is guided by means of an ultrasound monitor though the vagina and cervix. (A less frequently used approach is through the pelvic wall, with ultrasound guidance.) A small amount of tissue is suctioned from the placenta surrounding the baby and the sample cells are evaluated in a laboratory for the presence of certain problems.

How Accurate Is the Test?

CVS is a new test, but most experts feel that it is virtually as accurate as amniocentesis for the screening of many abnormalities such as Down's syndrome.

Since the cells are taken from the placenta and not the amniotic sac, occasionally a rare disorder may be missed, but improved techniques should cut down the possibility of this occurring.

What Are the Dangers of the Test?

Some initial studies reported a rate of 4 percent miscarriage following CVS. But these studies were poorly controlled and did not fully consider the normally increased rate of early miscarriage in the populations that were studied. More recent research shows that the dangers are between 1 and 2 percent, roughly equal to that of amniocentesis.

Where and by Whom Should the Test Be Performed and Interpreted?

Chorionic villus sampling can be performed in the doctor's office, or at a clinic or hospital. The procedure should be performed and the sample evaluated by an expert.

Is It Really Necessary?

Chorionic villus sampling may be appropriate during certain high-risk pregnancies:

- Women over the age of 35
- Women who have a history of many miscarriages
- Women who have previously given birth to children with genetic problems or have a family history of such problems

If you are pregnant, and think you may need prenatal diagnosis, you may want to compare amniocentesis and CVS.

THE ADVANTAGES AND DISADVANTAGES OF CVS AND AMNIOCENTESIS

1. The tests are roughly equal in accuracy and safety. However, CVS is a newer test, and the long-term complication rate has not yet been fully studied.
2. Only amniocentesis can diagnose certain nervous system problems, or fetal maturity and health late in pregnancy.
3. CVS may not be performed by the vaginal route if you have an active vaginal herpes infection or uterine fibroids.
4. CVS can be done eight weeks earlier than amniocentesis, and the results are usually available within days, rather than weeks.

The decision to abort is an individual one fraught with religious and moral controversy. The discussion of the pros and cons of abortion is beyond the scope of this book. If abortion is undertaken for medical reasons, however, the earlier timing of CVS should be considered, since abortions are safer and easier to carry out early in pregnancy.

TWO OTHER PRENATAL TESTS

Alfa-fetoprotein (AFP)

The testing of a prospective mother's blood for this substance may indicate the presence of certain defects in the unborn baby. Low levels may indicate Down's syndrome and high levels may suggest spina bifida.

But its use as a routine screening test has been the subject of heated controversy.

In 1982, the American College of Obstetrics and Gynecology (ACOG) stated that the test should be performed only when full diagnostic workup can follow. This may include other blood tests, amniocentesis and/or ultrasound. ACOG has not changed that stance, but new methods for measuring the levels were approved in 1984, and a few states have passed laws requiring that it be offered to all pregnant women. Some experts argue that such rules should not be imposed by organizations outside medicine; others disagree. The controversy arises from the difficulty in interpreting test results.

Only 25 to 35 percent of fetuses with Down's syndrome may be identified with this test. That means that it will *miss nearly 75 percent,* and although 1 out of 1,000 live births do have spina bifida or some related nervous system problem, the test cannot assure diagnosis. For those reasons, use the following guidelines when considering the test:

1. If you have a high-risk pregnancy—you're over the age of 35, or have a personal or family history of Down's syndrome—discuss the test with your doctor.
2. If you do undergo the test, make sure that you realize its limitations, and make sure that other tests, such as amniocentesis or chorionic villus sampling, are considered as well, before a final diagnosis is made.

Routine Ultrasound During Pregnancy

Ultrasound examinations are regularly performed during pregnancies in Europe, whether or not the pregnancy is considered "high-risk," but the procedure has not received widespread endorsement in the United States. Although it's considered safe by most experts, some doctors worry that its accuracy in the diagnosis of Down's syndrome and other developmental problems has not yet been sufficiently proven to warrant its routine use. For the time being, therefore, use the following guidelines regarding the performance of ultrasound during your pregnancy:

1. If you and your baby are at risk because you are over age 35, have a personal or family history of fetal abnormalities, or a history of many miscarriages, discuss the need for ultrasound with your doctor.
2. If you do have an ultrasound test for any of those reasons, or decide on a "routine" test which then produces results that raise the possibility of an abnormality, make sure you consider the need for other, more specific diagnostic tests such as amniocentesis or CVS.

If your doctor suggests that you have one of these tests done, review its description here and ask our Six Crucial Questions before proceeding.

Although they can expose you to unnecessary danger and cost when they're performed for the wrong reasons, they can mean the difference between life and death for you and/or your unborn children when they are selected appropriately.

Tests for women are also included in Chapter Ten (Fertility Tests), Chapter Fifteen (Tests for Sexually Transmitted Diseases), and Chapter Seventeen (Home Medical Tests).

NINE

Tests for Men

Men, like women, have their own set of medical problems.

- Problems of the prostate gland affect nearly 30 percent of men in the course of their lives.
- One out of 11 men develops cancer of the prostate.
- Heart disease is far more prevalent in men than women before the age of fifty.
- Bladder cancer is nearly twice as common in men as it is in women.

Just as with women, early detection of these problems can lead to cure. Because of anatomical and genetic differences, however, there are a number of diagnostic tests which are unique to men, and some of the routine screening tests are used with different frequency and according to different guidelines than with women.

RECTAL EXAMS FOR PROSTATE PROBLEMS

What Is the Purpose of the Test?

Rectal examinations are performed to check for rectal growths, hemorrhoids, blood in the stool, and for the detection of prostate abnormalities in men.

How Is the Test Performed?

The doctor will ask you to bend over or lie on your side on the examination table. He will then insert a surgically gloved finger into your rectum, examine your prostate, and take a stool sample to test for blood. If he is checking for prostate infection, the exam may be done after you provide a sample of urine, and the doctor may "massage" your prostate before you provide a second sample.

Where and by Whom Should the Test Be Performed and Interpreted?

The test can be done in your doctor's office, at a clinic, in the hospital, or at home. Your primary-care physician can do the initial screening exam, but if he feels any suspicious areas, he may want it to be evaluated by a proctologist if the problem is in your intestine or a urologist if it is your prostate.

How Accurate Is the Test?

The rectal examination is considered to be among the most accurate early screening tests for the diagnosis of rectal and prostate problems. However, it will not yield an absolute diagnosis with regard to the cause of any of these problems, and it can miss the more subtle abnormalities.

Any positive finding should be evaluated and made more specific by other tests, such as transrectal ultrasound (see below), sigmoidoscopy (see page 148), and/or biopsy (see Chapter Twelve).

Negative findings in high-risk people (see below, "Is It Really Necessary?") or in the presence of symptoms may have to be rechecked or investigated further.

What Are the Dangers of Doing the Test?

If the test is done properly, gently and with a gloved hand, there are no dangers.

Is It Really Necessary?

The American Cancer Society (ACS) recommends that every man over the age of 40 have a yearly rectal exam. If you have a family or personal history of prostate or intestinal cancer, or you develop any symptoms such as blood in the stool, difficulty with urination, or pain around the bladder or rectum, you may have to have an exam earlier than 40, and more frequently than once a year.

TRANSRECTAL ULTRASOUND

What Is the Purpose of the Test?

Transrectal ultrasound is a noninvasive test that is currently used to follow the treatment or progression of prostate cancer. In the future, it will probably be used along with rectal examination to aid in the early detection of prostate abnormalities.

How Is the Test Performed?

The test is done while you lie on an examination table. Using the ultrasound monitor for guidance, your doctor will pass a small sound transducer into your rectum. The instrument will bounce sound waves against your intestine and prostate, then pick up their echos for transmission onto the monitor.

Where and by Whom Should the Test Be Performed and Interpreted?

The test can be performed in a doctor's office, a clinic, or hospital. It should be done and evaluated by a specialist—in most cases a urologist or a specialized radiologist who has experience with the procedure.

How Accurate Is the Test?

Transrectal ultrasound is still in its infancy, but it is considered highly accurate for the detection of prostate tumors. Its accuracy for diagnosing other problems has not yet been adequately studied.

What Are the Dangers of Doing the Test?

The test may cause some pain and minimal bleeding, but it should be safe otherwise.

Is It Really Necessary?

This is not a routine test. Initially, it was used only as a follow-up after a diagnosis of prostate cancer had been made, but most experts feel that it will eventually be recommended on a regular basis for certain high-risk men:

- Those with a history of prostate cancer
- Those with suspicious findings on rectal examination
- Those with a family or personal history of other prostate problems

A NOTE ABOUT URINARY PROBLEMS IN MEN

Unlike women, men do not develop urinary symptoms very frequently. The male anatomy makes infections of the bladder and kidney less likely. But because men may develop prostate infections, and because cancer of the bladder is much more common in men than in women, most experts recommend that you follow certain guidelines for the early detection of these diseases:

- See the doctor anytime you develop blood in the urine or difficulty urinating.
- If prostate infection is suspected, make sure that your urine is tested before and after rectal examination and prostate massage.
- Although men will develop symptoms of a sexually transmitted disease (STD) more often than women, any STD can occur without causing symptoms. See the doctor anytime you discover that you have been exposed to venereal diseases, whether or not you have symptoms.

See also sections on home tests for problems of erection (page 239), urinary tract infection (page 238), fertility testing (Chapter 10), testing for venereal disease (Chapter Fifteen), testicular self-examination (page 56), breast examination in the man (page 51), and tests for prostate infection (page 192).

TEN
Fertility Tests

A few years ago, I was consulted by a woman who was having trouble becoming pregnant. She and her husband had been trying for four years; he was 41 years old, she was 40. They had already spent nearly two thousand dollars on fertility tests. No cause for their inability to conceive had been found.

On further questioning, however, I discovered that only the woman had been tested. I referred them to a top fertility expert who made the diagnosis after a few inexpensive procedures. He determined that the man's sperm was "incompatible" with the woman's cervical mucus and solved the problem by washing the sperm with special chemicals (see page 142). The couple gave birth to a healthy boy a little more than a year later.

They were delighted, but they would have saved themselves a great deal of time and money if they had been aware of three simple facts about infertility:

- One out of every six couples in the United States is infertile, meaning that they are unable to conceive a child after a year of trying.
- More than 50 percent of all fertility problems are attributable, at least in part, to the male.
- The majority of fertility problems can be cured.

Whenever a fertility problem exists, both members of the couple should be evaluated. In order to understand fertility testing, you need first to understand how normal pregnancy occurs. During intercourse, healthy sperm—defined as being high in number, motile, and potent, or able to penetrate the egg—enter the cervix and swim through the uterus into the fallopian tubes. There they meet a healthy egg and penetrate and fertilize it. The resulting embryo moves down the tube to the wall of the uterus, where it implants itself and causes a change in hormonal balance. This change allows the embryo to remain in the womb and grow into a normal, healthy child. A problem with any of these processes can cause infertility.

Fertility testing may need to evaluate each step:

- *Semen analysis* evaluates the number, size, motility, and health of the sperm.
- *Postcoital tests* examine the sperm's compatibility with the woman's cervical mucus.
- *"Hamster" tests* evaluate the sperm's ability to penetrate the egg.
- *Blood tests for hormone levels* check the man's ability to make sperm, and the woman's ability to produce and release eggs.
- *Hysterosalpingograms* examine a woman's uterus and fallopian tubes to determine whether there's any scarring present.
- *Basal body temperature and ultrasound* examinations evaluate the woman's ability to ovulate and release healthy eggs.
- *Laparoscopies,* in extreme circumstances, evaluate the anatomy of the woman's reproductive tract to determine whether mechanical problems are causing the infertility.
- *Endometrial tissue sampling* evaluates the ability of the woman's uterus to accept a healthy embryo.

THE FERTILITY WORKUP FOR THE MAN

Semen Analysis

The fertility of a man's semen is determined by the number of sperm present: their health, their motility, their compatibility with the woman's cervical mucus, and their ability to penetrate the egg.

What Is the Purpose of the Test?

A semen analysis examines all these features of the man's semen, to discover which, if any, are causing the couple's infertility.

How Is the Test Performed?

The man will be asked to masturbate and deposit a specimen of his semen into a sterile container provided by the doctor. This sample will then be examined under a microscope in a lab, and tested for its volume, the number of sperm (sperm count), their shape, and motility.

Where and by Whom Should the Test be Performed and Interpreted?

The sample can be obtained either in the doctor's office or at home. If obtained at home, it should be protected from extreme heat, sunlight or cold, and it should reach the laboratory within an hour.

The doctor who examines and interprets the test should be either a gynecologist or a urologist trained in fertility testing.

How Accurate Is the Test?

Regarding the number, motility, and potency of sperm, the test is very accurate.

However, if the test reveals that the man's sperm *is* the cause of the couple's infertility, further testing may have to be done to determine what is interfering with the sperm's production or release (see "Is It Really Necessary?" below).

What Are the Dangers of Doing the Test?

There are no dangers to semen analysis.

Is It Really Necessary?

If a couple is unable to conceive, semen analysis should be among the first screening tests performed.

If this analysis shows abnormal results, blood tests (for hormone levels) and other, more invasive tests that evaluate a man's reproductive organs may be necessary.

If the results of semen analysis are normal, the next step may be a postcoital semen analysis.

Postcoital Semen Analysis

The couple will be instructed to have intercourse a few days before the expected date of the woman's ovulation, and a pelvic exam will be performed within a few hours to obtain a sample of the woman's cervical mucus. Examination of this fluid will provide information about the compatibility of sperm and mucus.

If they are compatible, a "hamster test" may be done on the sperm to determine whether it is able to penetrate an egg.

If there's a problem with penetration or if the sperm and mucus are incompatible, shown by a significant decrease in fertile sperm within the mucus, or by the presence of antibodies to the sperm, special chemical "washing" of the man's sperm and/or subsequent placement of it through the cervix into the uterus may help the couple to conceive.

FERTILITY WORKUP FOR THE WOMAN

Ovulation Testing

The woman's fertility tests begin with an evaluation of her ability to ovulate. Basal body temperature measurements are the oldest and simplest method, and new home testing kits now available allow you to perform the testing in the privacy of your home (see Chapter Seventeen). If these fail to yield an answer, pelvic ultrasound (see pages 126 and 133) and/or laparoscopy (page 146) may be necessary. If ovulation is normal, a hysterosalpingogram may be suggested.

Hysterosalpingogram

What Is the Purpose of the Test?

Hysterosalpingograms are performed to identify blockage, scarring, or other problems in the uterus or fallopian tubes that might interfere with conception. They can also be used to identify suspected uterine problems that may be causing miscarriages or very painful menstrual periods.

How Is the Test Performed?

Hysterosalpingograms are performed during a pelvic exam. A hollow tube is passed through the cervix into the uterus and a small quantity of dye is injected. The movement of this dye through the uterus and fallopian tubes is then monitored on an x-ray screen.

Where and by Whom Should the Test be Performed and Interpreted?

This test is normally done in a hospital or clinic. It should be performed and interpreted by an obstetrician–gynecologist or radiologist.

How Accurate Is the Test?

The test is extremely accurate for the diagnosis of blockage in the fallopian tubes.

What Are the Dangers of Doing the Test?

There is a 1 to 3 percent risk of infection following this test, which, although it is small, is higher than that of many of the other fertility tests.

Is It Really Necessary?

Since the risk is slightly more than with many other fertility procedures, hysterosalpingograms should be delayed until the other tests have been tried. If they are unable to provide a diagnosis, the hysterosalpingogram may show fallopian tube scarring to be the cause of infertility. Many of the new fertility techniques such as in vitro fertilization (the "test-tube-baby" procedure) or gamete intrafallopian transfer (the "GIFT" procedure) may enable the doctor to bypass the scarring and help the couple to conceive.

Because of technological leaps in fertility diagnosis and treatment, it is now possible for more than half of the couples who were formerly diagnosed as infertile to become parents.

Most of these tests are safe and painless.

If you have a problem conceiving, make sure to see a fertility expert—you may achieve the same joyous results as the couple described at the beginning of this chapter.

ELEVEN
Endoscopies: Using Tubes and Microscopes to Look Inside the Body

Endoscopy, which means the "examination of the inside," is used for the diagnosis and treatment of a wide variety of medical problems.

WHAT IS THE PURPOSE OF ENDOSCOPY?

Endoscopies are performed to diagnose and treat problems within a body location, without exposing you to the dangers of general surgery. Chronic pain, in a joint or the pelvis for example, is one reason for an endoscopy, as is the removal of small chips of bone fragment from an injured joint. Many of the new fertilization procedures are performed with a type of endoscopy called laparoscopy, and both the diagnosis and treatment of abnormal uterine bleeding may be carried out with hysteroscopy.

HOW ARE ENDOSCOPIES PERFORMED?

First you are given either general anesthesia or local numbing medication and sedation. A small incision is then made over the area to be examined, and a fine fiberoptic tube is inserted. In certain endoscopies the procedure is different. In upper gastrointestinal endoscopy the tube is swallowed, and in sigmoidoscopy, it is inserted through the rectum. These tubes are thin, flexible optical filaments along which light can travel and bend. You may have seen a "spray" of them in the "light bouquets" that you can purchase at lighting or novelty stores. Their ability to bend light and enable a doctor to see around corners is largely responsible for the success of endoscopies. The tubes contain microscopes and instruments that enable your doctor to view the inside of the area studied, take samples, and if necessary, provide treatment.

WHERE AND BY WHOM SHOULD ENDOSCOPY BE PERFORMED AND INTERPRETED?

Most endoscopies are performed in a hospital setting, though a very few may be performed in a doctor's office or clinic. They must be performed and interpreted by a doctor who is an expert both in endoscopy and in the field of medicine that deals with the area being studied.

Thus, joint arthroscopies should be done by orthopedic surgeons, and hysteroscopies, on the uterus, should be done by gynecologists.

HOW ACCURATE ARE THESE TESTS?

Since they provide direct viewing of the area being evaluated, they are extremely accurate for diagnosis of many problems. Because the scopes are small, however, an occasional problem may be missed and further tests may be necessary.

WHAT ARE THE DANGERS OF DOING THESE TESTS?

Endoscopies are *less* dangerous than general surgery, but, because they are invasive—they involve the invasion of your body with an instrument—they are *more* dangerous than noninvasive tests. The exact danger depends on the experience of the person performing the endoscopy, the area being worked on, and whether or not general anesthesia, which is more dangerous than local anesthesia, is used.

ARE ENDOSCOPIES REALLY NECESSARY?

Endoscopies are rarely routine or even first-line tests. Because they may carry some risk, they should be reserved for those problems that the less dangerous tests cannot diagnose. However, because they are safer than general surgery, and can also treat many problems that they or the less invasive tests do diagnose, there are many circumstances under which endoscopy is the appropriate choice.

TYPES OF ENDOSCOPY

Upper Gastrointestinal (G.I.) Endoscopy (Stomach and Esophagus)

You are awake for this endoscopy. An intravenous line is placed in one of your arm veins, you'll be given some sedating medication, and a small amount of local numbing medicine will be sprayed on the back of your throat to prevent the gag reflex.

As you lie on your side, you'll swallow the endoscopy tube until it reaches your stomach. The doctor will follow its progress on a special monitor.

The test is slightly uncomfortable and may be frightening, but the diameter of the tube is usually smaller than a bite-sized piece of food, and it rarely causes any pain. The doctor then uses the microscope within the tube to view the lining of your stomach and esophagus for signs of irritation, ulcer, tumor, or other medical problem. He can also take samples for study and give medication or other treatment (such as cautery, sealing with heat or another agent, to stop bleeding) through the endoscope.

If your endoscopy was elective (not for emergency treatment of bleeding ulcers, for instance), you're usually able to leave the hospital the same day, and complications from this procedure are rare—less than 0.1 percent.

The test is not routine, but it may be necessary to evaluate persistent abdominal pain, hiatal hernia, ulcer, difficulty swallowing, or unexplained vomiting, and to rule out cancer in an ulcer that fails to heal.

Laparoscopy

Laparoscopy, the insertion of an endoscopic tube into the abdominal and pelvic areas, has revolutionized the treatment of many gynecological and abdominal problems.

After you receive general anesthesia, the doctor will make a small incision near your belly button and insert the tube. Then, he'll use the fiberoptic microscope to examine abdominal and pelvic organs, take tissue samples, and perform delicate surgery.

The procedure is usually performed in a hospital operating room and should be carried out by a specially trained gynecologist or surgeon. Since a general anesthesia is used, it is slightly more dangerous than stomach endoscopy. Also the risk of infection is slightly higher because of the incision required. Overall, complications are rare—less than 4 in 1,000.

Laparoscopy, like any endoscopy, should not be used lightly. It is invasive, and other tests and treatments may need to be tried first. However, if those fail, or when minor surgery is needed, it is appropriate in the following situations:

- To diagnose and treat unexplained pelvic pain. In many cases, this includes the definitive diagnosis of endometriosis, a painful condition caused when pieces of uterine tissue grow in unusual sites within the abdominal cavity.
- To diagnose and possibly treat tubal or "ectopic" pregnancies (those that occur outside the uterus), infections, cysts, and small growths. Treatments may be carried out with a scalpel or with a laser.
- To infuse medication for the treatment of cancer or certain infections directly into the affected site.
- To diagnose the cause of female infertility and to perform various fertilization procedures.

Hysteroscopy

Hysteroscopy is a new procedure whereby the endoscope is inserted through a woman's cervix in order to examine the inside lining of her uterus. It may be done in a doctor's office, a clinic, or a hospital, without the use of general anesthesia. Many experts feel that it will one day replace dilatation and curettage for the diagnosis and treatment of certain gynecological problems. Believed to be less dangerous than D&C and possibly more accurate, it offers direct viewing of the area to be diagnosed and/or treated.

Currently, hysteroscopy is used to diagnose and treat abnormal uterine bleeding, and small fibroids, infections, or cysts that lie within the uterine cavity. It cannot be used to treat larger growths, and although it may be used to identify a cancer, most experts advise against its use in the treatment of that disease, since the scope is small and limited in its reach.

A Note About Dilatation & Curettage Procedure (D&C's)

D&Cs are among the most frequently performed operations in the United States. They're done by using progressively larger instruments to dilate the cervix, then scraping the inner lining of the uterus.

The procedure does not involve direct viewing of the area to be diagnosed and/or treated. Because of its "blind" nature, it is slightly more dangerous and less accurate than the newer endoscopies, and it has sometimes been criticized for its widespread use. It will continue to hold a place in medical diagnosis and treatment, however. Even though the newer techniques such as hysteroscopy may replace it for the diagnosis and treatment of some problems, the D&C may continue to be used for some others, including the cleaning out of the uterus after partial miscarriage.

Cystoscopy

Cystoscopy is the name of the endoscopy procedure that doctors use to examine the inside of the bladder. The doctor will give you medication to sedate you and numb your genital area, then pass the cystoscope through your urethra (the tube that transports urine from your bladder to the outside) into your bladder, where diagnosis and/or treatment are undertaken.

The procedure is uncomfortable, but will not cause undue pain if it's performed properly. The minor risk of infection can be reduced by using appropriate sterile procedures and antibiotics before, during, and after the cystoscopy. This endoscopy cannot be done while you have an active infection of the bladder, urethra, or genital area, as the infection could easily be spread. It is not a first-line test (other less complicated tests should be done first), but may be necessary to evaluate the cause of chronic pain or difficulty urinating, persistent urinary tract infections, unexplained blood in the urine, or to follow the course and treatment of bladder cancer.

Endoscopies of the Large Intestine: Proctoscopy, Sigmoidoscopy, and Colonoscopy

These procedures may save your life. According to the ACS, cancer of the large intestine is the second-leading cause of cancer deaths in the United States. If the guidelines for early detection methods, including these special endoscopies, were followed properly, 45,000 more people would be cured of the disease every year. The tests are all performed in much the same manner: in the hospital, clinic, or doctor's office. The only difference among them is the length of the tube—colonoscopes are the longest, proctoscopes the shortest—and the indications for having the procedure done.

Proctoscopies and sigmoidoscopies—from "sigmoid," the section of the intestine immediately above the colon—may be performed by your family doctor, an internist who specializes in problems of the intestine, or a general surgeon. Colonoscopies should be performed by one of the latter two who has experience with the colonoscope.

In each case, you might need to prepare for the test by altering your diet and taking certain medications. For colonoscopy, you may be asked to drink a few liters of saltwater before the test, or follow a liquid diet for a few days followed by laxatives the night before and an enema on the morning of the test. People who cannot handle a large salt load, such as those with heart disease or high blood pressure, may be forced to choose the second option. Proctoscopies and sigmoidoscopies may require only a brief liquid diet and laxatives the night before and/or a small enema on the day of the test. In either case, a clean intestine is essential for a good examination, so follow the instructions carefully.

You'll remain awake while you are given sedatives and local numbing medications. As you lie on your side, the doctor will slowly insert the lubricated endoscope into your rectum. He'll then view the inside of your rectum through the microscope as he advances the tube and follows its progress on an x-ray monitor. If he discovers any abnormalities, he may take tissue samples for study. Polyps may be removed entirely with the scope, although further surgery may be required if they are cancerous.

You may experience some bloating and pressure during the tests, but if they're done properly, they will not cause severe pain. The dangers of complications, such as bleeding or infection, are small—less than 0.01 percent for proctoscopy and sigmoidoscopy, 0.1 percent for colonoscopy.

Sigmoidoscopy is now suggested as a routine test by the ACS for people over the age of 50. You should have one every year after that age until two consecutive exams are normal, and every three to five years thereafter. If you have a personal or family history of diseases of the large intestine or develop symptoms such as blood in the stool, change in bowel regularity, or size and consistency of stool, the exams may have to be done sooner and more frequently.

Colonoscopies are more complex than are proctoscopies and sigmoidoscopies, and they are usually not considered routine.

However, since they allow the doctor to evaluate the entire large intestine rather than just the lower 1/4 or 1/3 that is examined with sigmoidoscopy, they may be recommended in the following circumstances:

- When symptoms such as abdominal pain or blood in the stool exist, and sigmoidoscopy, proctoscopy, and barium enema (see page 166) fail to yield a diagnosis
- When a barium enema reveals an abnormality that the sigmoidoscope cannot reach
- When a person is discovered (by barium enema or sigmoidoscopy) to have cancer of the large intestine, to check and make sure that no other areas of cancer exist and to follow the patient's progress regularly after surgery.
- For the patient with "familial polyposis," a disease that causes the development of numerous polyps and increases the risk of intestinal cancer

A recent study suggested that colonoscopies may miss or fail to localize a cancer if done without a previous or ensuing barium enema. Therefore, whenever the tests are indicated for diagnosis or to follow the course of a patient with a previous cancer, they may be thought of as complementary.

According to the ACS, the current five-year survival rate of people with cancer of the large intestine is 55 percent—but this could be increased to 85 percent if we all followed the guidelines regarding rectal exams (page 55), tests of the stool for blood (page 236), and these endoscopies of the large intestine.

Bronchoscopy

Bronchoscopy is the endoscopic procedure used for the examination of the inside of your breathing passages and lungs. It is usually performed by an internist who specializes in lung problems or by a chest surgeon, in an office, clinic, or hospital.

You remain awake, but gently sedated, while the doctor sprays the back of your throat with an anesthetic solution to prevent the gag reflex, then inserts a fiberoptic tube through your nose or mouth into your trachea and bronchi, the main air passages into your lungs.

The doctor views the condition of your airways, collects tissue samples, and may give you medication or wash out some of these airways with a saline solution.

The test may be frightening and uncomfortable, but should not be painful. It may carry some risk, however: the most common complication is pneumonia, which some studies say occurs in as many as 4 percent of people who have the test. Also, when large tissue samples are taken, collapse of a small part of the lung has been reported 2 percent of the time. Both of these problems are usually treated without serious consequence, and other, more serious complications are rare, occurring in less than 0.2 percent of patients.

Bronchoscopy is not a routine test, but it may be indicated under the following circumstances:

- To diagnose a tumor, infection, or other lung problem that has been discovered but incompletely evaluated by a chest x-ray or other test
- To diagnose the cause of unexplained, persistent cough, blood in the sputum, or wheezing and shortness of breath
- To deliver certain medications
- To remove foreign objects or excessive secretions
- For minor surgery on tumors or abscesses

Arthroscopy

Arthroscopy makes use of a tiny endoscope to examine the inside of your joints. Most frequently performed by an orthopedic surgeon in an operating room, it has made the repair of many joint problems possible without the dangers of major surgery.

Since general anesthesia is often given, the procedures carry the slight increase in danger associated with its use (the risk of serious reaction to general anesthesia is about 0.3 percent) but they are otherwise relatively safe. Complications such as joint infections and bleeding into the joint occur in less than 0.1 percent of cases.

After the anesthesia has taken effect, a small incision is made over the joint so that the fiberoptic tube can be inserted into the joint space. A small quantity of saline solution may be injected via the arthroscope to expand the joint and provide a clearer picture of what is going on. The inside of the joint is then examined through the microscope and diagnosis and treatment are undertaken. The knee was the first joint to be examined and treated with the arthroscope, but recent developments in fiberoptics have made arthroscopies possible on the ankle, hip, shoulder, wrist, and elbow as well.

Possible indications for arthroscopy are the following:

- To diagnose chronic joint pain that has not been explained by less invasive tests such as x-ray, CAT scan, or MRI
- To view joints that are unstable or have had their range of motion decreased by injury
- To confirm a diagnosis obtained from a physical exam, x-ray or arthrogram (the x-ray of a joint that has been stained with dye)
- To remove small pieces of chipped bone, shave a bone to improve motion, or remove a foreign body

Endoscopies represent a major step forward in health care. Through the use of fiberoptic filaments and microscopic surgical instruments, they make possible the treatment of many medical conditions that would otherwise require major surgery. In cases where endoscopies can't be used to solve a problem, they can improve diagnosis and increase the chances for success of subsequent surgery.

TWELVE
Taps, Biopsies, and Cultures

TAPS

What Is the Purpose of the Tests?

Taps are done to determine whether fluid has collected in a body space, to diagnose the cause of the collection, to relieve suffering, and/or to inject medication.

How Are Taps Performed?

A tap is a procedure where the doctor uses a needle to remove fluid from a joint or other body space.

It is done while you are awake. First the doctor numbs the area with Novocaine or a similar anesthetic, then he inserts the needle and withdraws the fluid.

Where and by Whom Should the Tests Be Performed and Interpreted?

Taps can be done in a clinic, an office, or a hospital. They can be performed and interpreted by any primary-care physician, but when diagnosis or treatment is in doubt, a specialist may be necessary. For instance, you may want an orthopedist to do a joint tap, unless it's for the simple removal of fluid in an injured knee for relief of pain caused by the pressure of fluid buildup, in which case any doctor with experience can perform the test. Similarly, you may prefer a lung doctor for a lung tap, or a surgeon for an abdominal tap.

How Accurate Are the Tests?

Taps are extremely accurate for the diagnosis of infection and crystals.

The diagnosis of cancer with a tap may prove more difficult. Cancer can cause fluid to accumulate in an area, but the needle may miss the cells, thereby missing the diagnosis. Usually, this problem can be overcome by analyzing the fluid for other characteristics indicative of cancer.

What Are the Dangers of the Tests?

Taps generally carry a slight risk of infection in the area studied and of localized bleeding. Certain taps, such as those involving the lung or heart, may be more dangerous, since a slip of the needle could harm an important organ. You can reduce the dangers by making sure that an expert performs the test.

Are the Tests Really Necessary?

Taps are rarely first line tests and they are never routine. They may be necessary when simple tests like x-rays, blood tests or other "non-invasive" procedures do not produce a diagnosis, or if fluid needs to be removed to relieve pain or suffering. One such example is the removal of fluid from the "pleural" areas around the lung in a patient with cancer or infection. This is done to make it easier for him or her to breathe.

TYPES OF COMMON TAPS

Abdominal

Abdominal taps are used for the diagnosis of injury, infection, or cancer.

Pleural (Around the Lung Area)

Pleural taps are used for diagnosis or for the relief of pressure and difficulty in breathing.

Cardiac (Heart)

Cardiac taps are usually used as a life-saving measure to remove fluid that has accumulated around the heart, as can happen in conditions such as "pericarditis" or "pericardial tamponade." A cardiac tap may occasionally be used for diagnosis of infection or other heart problems.

Spinal

Spinal taps are now used mainly for the diagnosis of infection of the spinal cord and brain such as meningitis. Although taps formerly were used to diagnose brain hemorrhage such as occurs with "subdural hematomas" or "subarachnoid bleeding" from burst aneurysms, they have since been replaced by the safer, less invasive CAT scans and MRI's for those purposes.

Joint

Joint taps are used for the diagnosis of infection, injury, inflammation, or cancer and to distinguish among rheumatoid, infectious, and gout arthritis.

A tap may also be used to relieve the pain caused by accumulated fluid or to inject medication directly into a joint.

Culdocentesis

Culdocentesis is used for the diagnosis of pelvic pain in women. In this procedure, the doctor inserts a needle into the wall of the vagina behind the cervix and withdraws fluid for study. Culdocentesis can assist in the detection of tubal pregnancies, bleeding, and infection. However, it is usually performed only when ultrasound and other noninvasive tests have failed to yield a diagnosis.

BIOPSIES

Biopsies are performed to obtain cells or tissue for direct examination.

What Is the Purpose of the Test?

Biopsies are used to determine the cause of unexplained diseases, swelling, masses, and tumors.

How Is the Test Performed?

If the doctor wishes to biopsy a mole or some similar tissue on the skin, he will numb the area with an injection of Novocaine, then simply scrape or remove the tissue with a scalpel.

If the biopsy needs to be done on an organ such as the breast or liver, a hollow needle will be used to draw out a sample. Your doctor may use x-rays, ultrasound or other imaging techniques to ensure that the needle reaches the correct destination.

In rare circumstances, when the tissue to be biopsied is very deep within the body, or when your doctor suspects that major surgery to remove cancerous tissue may immediately follow the biopsy, you may require general anesthesia.

Where and by Whom Should the Test Be Performed and Interpreted?

Biopsies are usually performed by the specialist in the area in question: a lung specialist for lung biopsies, a hematologist (blood specialist) for bone marrow biopsies, an abdominal specialist for liver biopsies, and so on. Skin biopsies may be performed by a dermatologist, surgeon, or family physician. They should be interpreted by a pathologist who has experience in identifying tissues and cell types in that area of the body.

How Accurate Are the Tests?

Biopsies are extremely accurate when an adequate sample of tissue is obtained for study, as long as the sample is interpreted by the correct specialists.

What Are the Dangers of the Tests?

All biopsies are associated with a slight risk of local infection or bleeding. The more elaborate biopsies, such as those on liver, lung, or kidney, carry the increased danger of injury to a vital organ. You can decrease these risks by making sure that an expert with experience in biopsying that particular region does your test.

Is It Really Necessary?

Biopsy is the first-line test when a suspicious area is found on the skin, but when a lump, growth, or suspicious area is found within the body or on an organ, it may have to be first evaluated by noninvasive tests, such as x-ray, CAT scans, or MRI's. If these noninvasive tests don't yield an exact diagnosis, they'll help to define the area in question, reduce the dangers, and improve the accuracy of subsequent biopsy. Once they've been completed, the biopsy can provide the final, definitive diagnosis.

CULTURES

What Is the Purpose of the Test?

Cultures are done in order to detect the presence of an infecting organism, usually a bacterium.

Cultures may occasionally be used for the detection of viruses, fungi, and other organisms as well.

How Are Cultures Performed?

Cultures are done by using a sterile swab, scalpel, or needle to collect a specimen of fluid or tissue. This specimen is then "cultured," which means that bacteria present in the specimen are grown in a glass dish in a laboratory. This makes the bacteria cells easily identifiable. After the bacteria have been identified, they are tested for sensitivity to certain medications.

When blood is being cultured, up to four specimens may be necessary, taken from different veins and at different times. Cultures are also done on urine, the throat (to diagnose "strep throat"), wounds, fluid obtained from taps, stool, and sputum—material that is coughed up.

Where and by Whom Should the Test Be Performed and Interpreted?

Cultures can be performed by any trained laboratory technician. In certain circumstances, the technician is capable of interpreting the cultures, but if the diagnosis is at all unclear, he should seek the help of a physician who has experience in culture interpretation.

How Accurate Is the Test?

A culturer's accuracy depends on the technique, method of collection, and culture site. It is far more accurate when done carefully and by skilled personnel. Also, cultures of the urine or of obviously infected wounds are more accurate than those of joints or blood.

While certain viral cultures, such as the culture test for Herpes, have been improved in recent years, overall, bacterial cultures are much more accurate than most viral cultures. Still, even they are capable of missing a good number of organisms. For this reason, the diagnosis of infection must often be based on physical exam and history as well as on the results of a culture.

What Are the Dangers of the Test?

The only dangers associated with most cultures are the minor risks of bleeding or infection at the culture site. If blood cultures are not done properly, the additional risk of introducing further infection into the blood exists.

Are Cultures Really Necessary?

Cultures are not done routinely. However, any time an infection is suspected, a culture should be attempted, before antibiotics or other antimicrobial medications are prescribed. Treatment may have to begin before the results are available, but a properly performed culture can confirm or refute a diagnosis, help to guide later treatment, and, in some cases, can mean the difference between life and death.

Cultures may be appropriate for the following situations:

- On sore throats suspected of being caused by the streptococcus bacterium
- On infected wounds
- On urine when urinary symptoms such as frequency, burning on urination, or blood in the urine exist, or when back pain and fever exists and your doctor suspects a kidney infection
- On stool when persistent diarrhea exists and a bacterial infection is suspected
- On sputum when a lung infection is suspected
- On genital discharge or sores
- On blood when there is unexplained, persistent fever or a suspicion of drug abuse and/or infection of the heart valves ("endocarditis")
- On the spinal fluid obtained from a spinal tap when meningitis or some other infection of the nervous system is suspected
- On fluid obtained from other taps when an infection of a body space is suspected

Once medication is prescribed, the cultures may need to be repeated to improve the accuracy of the diagnosis, check on progress, and/or make sure that the infection is responding to the treatment.

Taps, biopsies, and cultures all carry the minor risks of localized infection and moderate discomfort. In certain cases, though, they can provide the definitive word on diagnosis and treatment. If your doctor suggests that you have one of these procedures performed, review its description above and make sure to discuss all Six Crucial Questions with him before having it done.

THIRTEEN

Imaging: Techniques That Give Us the Inside View Without the Use of Scalpels, Tubes, or Needles

Doctors have been trying to find a way to see inside the body without the use of scalpels and tubes since the practice of medicine began. The first such noninvasive imaging to be successful was the simple x-ray. It's ability to produce pictures of our internal organs has revolutionized medical care, and it remains an important tool today.

Yet, for all its value, the simple x-ray has disadvantages: it exposes us to potentially dangerous doses of radiation and produces only flat, two-dimensional pictures.

Dye studies took us a step further. They provide a more detailed look at our insides by combining a "radio-opaque" dye, one that shows up on x-ray film after being injected, swallowed, or introduced by enema, with simple x-rays. But they have some disadvantages as well: they're slightly more invasive than simple x-rays, they may carry an even greater risk of radiation exposure, and, for the most part, they're limited to the examination of hollow organs, such as our blood vessels, stomach, or intestine.

Nuclear scans were the first imaging technique to improve our diagnostic abilities without increasing the dangers. These tests are performed with radionuclides, very tiny doses of radioactive substances that emit energy. When they're injected, swallowed, or inhaled, they quickly move through the body and collect in various organs. Special monitors detect their energy and translate it into pictures that provide information about each organ not apparent on simple x-rays.

Ultrasound tests bounce sound waves off internal organs and translate the "echo" into amazingly clear images on televisionlike monitors. Although some scientists have speculated on the potential danger to the long-term effects of sound waves, no danger has been demonstrated, and most experts consider ultrasound completely safe. Making up nearly 15 percent of all imaging procedures, the technique is invaluable for the diagnosis of a wide variety of problems in many different parts of the body. Its success is more limited in people who are very overweight, or in areas where bone or gas, such as the large intestine, might interfere with the image.

CAT scans (computerized transaxial tomography), also called CT scans, were the next imaging technique to be developed, and many experts feel that they are among the most important diagnostic inventions of this century. They combine a moving x-ray machine with a computer to produce what doctors call "slices," images at precise depths within our bodies that enable us to see the inside of each organ as a series of layers.

Among the newest imaging technologies are SPECT (single photon emission computerized tomography—see page 181) and PET (positron emission tomography—see page 180). SPECT uses radionuclides in combination with CAT scanners to produce detailed moving pictures of these organs. PET scanners use substances that our bodies need and metabolize, such as sugar, that have been radioactively labeled so that they emit detectable energy. The migration of the substance through the body is followed, to provide information about the function of each organ.

MRI (Magnetic Resonance Imaging) uses a giant magnet to shake up the body's atoms and create precise, detailed pictures of the inside of the body without the use of injections or radiation.

These amazing imaging techniques have improved our ability to see inside of our bodies while decreasing the chances of pain or side effects. Because of their value and their almost science-fiction-like nature, they've gotten wide play in the media, but what you've seen or heard until now may have confused you. The names alone might make you feel as though you're dealing with a complex crossword puzzle, and you might think that it's impossible for you to understand the differences or to know which techniques are appropriate for you.

We'll make it easy.

Read through the description of each imaging technique. You'll learn exactly how each is performed, how it feels, and what information it can provide.

In the future, should your doctor suggest that you have one of these tests, you'll be able to consider its advantages, disadvantages, and risks before deciding whether or not to have it done. Most important, you'll know what your alternatives are.

SIMPLE X-RAYS

When Wilhelm Roentgen discovered the x-ray around the turn of the century, he probably had no idea that it would literally change the face of medicine. X-rays have been used for more than sixty years to aid in the diagnosis and treatment of disease. Today, despite concern about radiation exposure and the development of newer imaging tests, the simple x-ray still occupies an important place in medical practice.

What Is the Purpose of X-rays?

X-rays are performed to give your doctor a view of the inside of your body without cutting you open. Each x-ray is performed for its own reason: a bone x-ray might be used to detect a fracture or a tumor; a chest x-ray to check for infection, cancer, or emphysema.

How Is an X-ray Performed?

X-rays are made up of electromagnetic radiation. This radiation is generated by the x-ray machine and aimed at the part of your body being studied. You stand, sit, or lie between the machine and an x-ray film, which has been impregnated with silver nitrate. The x-ray beams pass through your body and each tissue absorbs different amounts.

The tissues, such as bone, that absorb the most appear whitest on the negative film; the tissues that absorb the least appear darkest.

Where and by Whom Should an X-ray Be Performed and Interpreted?

X-rays can be performed by licensed technicians in an office, a clinic, or a hospital. Your family doctor can probably interpret many different types of x-rays, but whenever he's unsure, or whenever the more advanced, specific techniques are used, they should be interpreted by a radiologist.

How Accurate Are the Tests?

X-rays are accurate but limited. They are really just like photographs, simple two-dimensional pictures of your insides. They pick up most clear, simple changes on the surface of internal organs, and an experienced doctor should be able to infer deeper problems from changes in the x-ray's appearance. They are not as accurate as three-dimensional pictures for picking up problems that require depth perception, for example, the exact location of a tumor or infection. Multiple views, such as a frontal and lateral chest x-ray, partially solve this problem, but many organs and diseases remain out of the simple x-ray's reading capacity.

Are X-rays Dangerous?

There's no question that exposure to radiation is potentially dangerous, but many experts believe that the doses used in diagnostic x-rays carry little risk, and that the dangers need to be seen in perspective.

Since x-rays have to be absorbed in order to produce different contrasts on the x-ray film, a certain amount of the electromagnetic radiation will remain in your tissues. "Rads" are the units used to express absorbed radiation. Each different type of x-ray exposes you to a different number of rads, depending on the voltage used and the number of films taken. Chest x-rays expose you to the least, certain dye studies the most.

The following is a list of various simple x-rays in *ascending* order of radiation exposure:

Low exposure   Chest, skull, long bone (arm or leg), and dental x-rays

Medium exposure   Abdominal, neck, certain dye studies including barium swallows, and coronary angiography

Higher exposure   Lower back, certain dye studies, including barium enemas, intravenous pyelograms (IVP's), and abdominal angiograms

Viewing these dangers in perspective means taking a number of other facts into consideration as well:

1. The radiation dose is cumulative over the course of a lifetime. For this reason you should have only x-rays that are essential for diagnosis. You should limit the number of x-rays to which your child is exposed.
2. X-rays in high doses and over a long period of time can represent a danger to your reproductive organs and you should protect them unless they lie in the area to be studied. If you are of child-bearing age,

make sure to cover them with a lead apron (which acts as a barrier to the rays) every time you have an x-ray.

3. Although you should remain constantly aware of each of these dangers and keep your x-ray exposure to a minimum, before rejecting the test, you should also consider the dangers of missing a diagnosis that could be provided by an x-ray.

4. You should realize that a simple chest x-ray exposes you to less radiation than one cross-country plane flight, or a car ride the length of California in a convertible.

Is It Really Necessary?

Only two types of x-ray are considered routine, chest x-rays for men and women at the age of 40 and 60, and mammograms for women—the first between the ages of 35 and 40, one every one to two years between 40 and 49, and one every year thereafter.

The value of using chest x-rays to screen for disease in healthy people has come under recent fire, but the value of mammograms for the early detection of breast cancer is unquestioned.

All other simple x-rays should be done only when the need arises, and after weighing the relative risks of getting the x-ray against the risks of skipping it.

When thinking about those factors, consider whether the results will change treatment.

Here are a few examples

- A repeat back x-ray, which exposes you to a high amount of radiation, for what your doctor is sure is muscle strain may not be worth the risk if your treatment will be the same no matter what it shows. It might be worth the risk if it will help your doctor decide whether or not you need surgery.

- X-rays of long bones expose you to low radiation; in the case of a leg or arm injury, the information they yield may help the doctor decide whether you need a cast, an ace bandage, or surgery.

- Studies have shown that skull x-rays, which also expose you to a low dose of radiation, are not necessary for all head injuries. They should be especially avoided in children, since radiation dosage is cumulative over a lifetime.

Don't assume that you will be able to avoid all x-rays, for they may occasionally be necessary. But don't be afraid to second-guess your doctor either.

Every time an x-ray is suggested, ask if the results might change your treatment. If they won't, you simply don't need the test. If they could, consider the amount of radiation exposure of that specific test—as well as what you've already been exposed to—and weigh those dangers against the need for the test before you decide. If you're still unsure, ask if one of the newer techniques might yield similar or better information while exposing you to less danger.

DYE STUDIES

What Is the Purpose of the Tests?

Dye studies produce pictures of the inside of hollow organs, such as the blood vessels or intestines. They are used to diagnose a blockage or an aneurysm (a weakness that causes a "ballooning" or enlargement) in an artery, a tumor in the large intestine or stomach, or an ulcer in the stomach or small intestine.

How Are the Tests Performed?

Dye studies are performed by injecting, inserting (as in barium enemas) or having you swallow a substance that shows up on an x-ray.

Where and by Whom Should the Tests Be Performed and Interpreted?

Some dye studies must be done in a hospital, others can be done in a clinic or a doctor's office. They should be performed and interpreted by a doctor who has experience in studying the area under examination or by a specialized radiologist.

How Accurate Are the Tests?

Dye studies are extremely accurate for the area studied. Angiograms show the clearest picture of blockage in blood vessels, and barium swallows and enemas, along with endoscopies, produce among the clearest images of changes in the esophagus, stomach, and intestine.

What Are the Dangers of the Tests?

The dangers depend on the specific test: those that involve injections carry the minimal risk of local infections or bleeding around the injection site. Heart or brain dye studies may carry more risk than other dye studies because of the sensitive nature of each of those organs.

Are They Really Necessary?

Dye studies are never routine. They are necessary whenever the inside of a tubelike organ, such as a blood vessel or the stomach, needs to be examined, and other less invasive tests have not produced a diagnosis. In certain cases, the dye study is the only way to make a definitive diagnosis. In others, there may be alternatives, such as radionuclide studies.

See the description of each test for its specific indications.

TYPES OF DYE STUDIES

Angiograms

Angiograms are performed by injecting a blood vessel with dye. If the blood vessel to be studied is an artery, the test is called an arteriogram, if it's a vein, it's called a venogram. Angiograms must be done in a hospital, and you will probably stay overnight. Angiograms are still the definitive tests for examining the anatomy of a blood vessel, and they may be used for other purposes as well, including identification of certain tumors and aneurysms.

Types of Angiograms

Abdominal   Study of the blood vessels that supply your abdominal organs.

Aortic   Study of the largest artery in your body, the aorta.

Cerebral   Study of the brain circulation.

Carotid   Study of the large blood vessels in your neck that bring blood to the brain.

Coronary   Study of the blood vessels that supply blood to the heart.

Lung   A recent study done by the National Heart, Lung and Blood Institute called lung (or pulmonary) angiograms "the definitive test" for pulmonary embolism, or blood clot in the lung. Like all angiograms, the pulmonary angiogram carries some risk, and may be superseded by the safer lung radionuclide scan (see page 170).

Kidney   May be used to check for tumors and other abnormalities.

Venograms   May be used to study the veins in your legs to check for blockage or clots.

Lymphangiograms   These are dye studies of the lymph vessels that connect your lymph nodes. They're usually performed by injecting dye into a small lymph vessel in your foot. Lymphangiograms are also used to study certain cancers of the lymph system, such as Hodgkin's disease.

Digital Subtraction Angiograms (DSA)   DSA is done by injecting dye into a blood vessel, then using a computer to subtract unwanted shadows that might obscure the view of the area being studied. The result is a clearer, more precise picture than is produced by regular angiography.

Some universities are already using DSA to visualize the heart and its blood vessels. Researchers believe it will be employed to study many other parts of the body in the course of the next decade.

Arthrogram

Arthrograms, which can be done in an office, clinic, or hospital, involve the injection of dye into a joint to study its structure and determine whether surgery is required to repair an injury. They may also be used to evaluate undiagnosed chronic joint pain.

Barium Enema

Barium enemas are most often performed to determine whether any cancers are present in the large intestine. They may be indicated if you have a change in bowel habits, a change in size or quality of your stool, or blood in the stool.

The tests are performed in a hospital or clinic by using an enema device to insert barium into your rectum. You're asked to "hold" this barium while x-rays are taken of your large intestine. Many people complain that the test is very uncomfortable, but not painful.

Sigmoidoscopy (see page 148) may precede this test, and it may save you from needing one, if it's able to detect the cause of your symptoms; in certain instances, colonoscopy may be also be necessary (see page 148). A recent study suggested that a colonoscopy may miss or fail to localize a cancer if done without a previous or ensuing barium enema. Therefore, whenever the tests are indicated for diagnosis or to follow the course of treatment of a patient with a previous cancer, colonoscopy and barium enema may be thought of as complementary.

Barium Swallow

During this test, you swallow a small amount of a chalklike substance called barium and x-rays are taken of your esophagus and stomach. If the small intestine is also studied, it's called an upper gastrointestinal series. The x-rays can detect activity in these organs, such as an abnormality in the peristalsis (swallowing action) of the esophagus, or to check for foreign bodies or blockages, tumors, or ulcers.

Cholecystograms (Gallbladder Tests)

Your gallbladder may be studied through the use of dye that is either swallowed—an oral cholecystogram—or injected—an intravenous cholecystogram.

You may be asked to eat a meal high in fats as part of the test, to see how your gallbladder reacts to a fat load. Whether or not you do this, your abdomen will be examined with multiple x-rays as the dye makes its way through the gallbladder. The procedure has, in the past, been performed to evaluate the possibilities of gallstones and other diseases of the gallbladder, but it is being replaced by ultrasound and other new and less invasive techniques.

Intravenous Pyelogram (IVP)

IVP's are done to study your kidneys for the presence of kidney stones, blockages, or chronic infections or to evaluate undiagnosed flank pain, changes in urinary habit, or blood in the urine.

An IVP is performed by injecting dye into one of the veins in your arm, then taking numerous x-rays as it passes through your kidneys.

Cystourethrogram

This test is performed to detect signs of injury to the urinary tract. Dye is injected into your urethra and through the urethra into your bladder, so both can be studied. A cystourethrogram may also be used along with an IVP to diagnose the cause of chronic infections or blood in the urine.

Myelogram

This test involves the injection of dye into your spinal cord, to help diagnose slipped discs, tumors, injuries, and other problems.

Because myelograms have resulted in some severe side effects, including life-threatening allergic reactions, they are usually reserved for patients who require surgery and in whom CAT scans or MRI's have been unable to provide all the necessary information.

RADIONUCLIDE SCANS

Radionuclide scans, such as Thallium or PET scans, employ a small amount of radionuactive substance to study your internal organs while they function.

What Is the Purpose of the Tests?

Scans are done to detect abnormalities in the various organs they study. One of their advantages over simple x-rays is that they can watch the organ while it moves and gather information about its performance and function as well as its anatomy. They can diagnose tumors, infections, changes in blood flow, and blockages.

How Are the Tests Performed?

A very small amount of a radioactive substance, called a radionuclide, is injected, inhaled, or swallowed. As this radionuclide passes through your body, it emits radiation and collects in various organs. A special monitor or scanner picks up the radiation and transforms it into what looks like a fuzzy television picture.

The organ being studied and the information being sought determine what type of radionuclide is used.

Where and by Whom Should the Scans Be Performed and Interpreted?

Radionuclide scans are the province of a whole new medical specialty called nuclear medicine. They are most often performed and interpreted in a hospital, by specialized radiologists or nuclear medicine specialists.

How Accurate Are the Tests?

The accuracy of scans depends on a number of factors: the organ being studied, the radionuclide itself, the conditions under which the scan is done, and the expert performing and interpreting the test. Thus a resting thallium scan of the heart may pick up a certain percentage of abnormalities when done alone, but it may pick up far more than when combined with a treadmill ("stress") thallium (see page 97). Since the tests are so complex, their interpretation may depend on correlation with your symptoms, physical exam, and other tests—all of which require an expert for evaluation.

What Are the Dangers of Scans?

Nuclear scans involve the same radiation danger as x-rays. In most cases the exposure is less, but because the reproductive organs can't be shielded as easily as with simple x-rays, many experts try to avoid these procedures with pregnant or breast-feeding women.

The radionuclide itself is completely eliminated from the body within days (sometimes, with PET scans, within minutes) and no adverse long-term effects have been reported to date. Nevertheless, the theoretical danger exists, and you should keep such exposure to a minimum.

Are Scans Really Necessary?

Nuclear scans represent a major step forward in medical diagnosis. They enable us to see organs while they function, with relatively few risks. These are rarely first-line tests, however. Radionuclide scans are expensive and complex, and should be used only when less complex tests have not produced a diagnosis. Under those circumstances, which depend on the organ being studied (see below), scans may provide invaluable information.

TYPES OF RADIONUCLIDE SCANS

With the exception of lung ventilation scans, which involve inhalation, the following tests all require that the substance be injected into a vein in one of your arms.

Bone Scan

Bone scans are done to diagnose chronic bone pain, to determine whether a bone infection (osteomyelitis) is present, or to detect bone cancer. They're often more accurate than simple x-rays for the detection of these problems, but the x-rays should almost always be done first, to determine whether a scan is needed.

Brain Scan

Brain scans were used in the past to detect tumors, infections, or other abnormalities of the brain, but CAT and MRI tests are now replacing them as the procedure of choice.

Gallium Scan

Gallium scans are used to evaluate problems that have not produced localizing symptoms, such as persistent, unexplained fever or generalized lymph node swelling. It is the only radionuclide scan that studies the entire body.

Although gallium scans may detect early signs of infection or certain cancers, they may miss many others. They are not very precise: since gallium is picked up by normal bone, liver, and other tissues, areas of increased uptake may be difficult to interpret. Therefore, gallium scans should not be used as a routine screening test. They are indicated only to follow the treatment of certain cancers, such as Hodgkin's disease, or for persistent, generalized problems that other tests have failed to diagnose.

Liver-Spleen Scan

Liver-spleen scans are usually performed to determine if either organ has been affected by cancer. They can also be used to evaluate an abdominal injury, unexplained abdominal pain, or enlargement of either organ.

Lung Scan

Lung scans are most often performed to determine if a blood clot has traveled to the lungs. Since these clots, called pulmonary embolisms, usually originate in the leg veins during a condition called thrombophlebitis, a lung scan may be ordered when you have thrombophlebitis and begin to experience chest pain or shortness of breath.

The scan is often done in two steps: ventilation and perfusion. In the ventilation part, you inhale the radioactive gas, and the monitor checks the lung for areas that do not receive air. During the perfusion scan, the radionuclide is injected, and the monitor checks for areas which don't receive blood.

Segments that receive air but not blood are considered to be blocked by a pulmonary embolism and treatment is begun, usually with medicines that break up the clot. Rarely, an embolectomy is performed (a procedure where a tube is inserted into the lung veins in an attempt to break up the clot) and, in life-threatening circumstances, surgery.

A lung scan is not a routine test, but it is appropriate when a diagnosis of a pulmonary embolism is being considered. Ventilation scans may be used alone to evaluate lung disease.

Scrotal Scans

Nuclear scans of the scrotum and testicles may provide crucial information in the treatment of severe scrotal pain.

Sudden onset of such pain may be due either to torsion, a twisting of the testicle requiring immediate surgery to save the testicle, or to an infection called epididymitis, which requires treatment with antibiotics.

The scan is performed by injecting the radionuclide into an arm vein and then scanning the scrotum with a special monitor. Since a doctor can differentiate between the two causes of pain with this scan, it may mean the difference between saving the testicle and losing it.

Thallium and Technetium Heart Scans

These scans are used to detect decreased blood flow to the heart, to determine if a blockage in flow in reversible, to aid in the diagnosis of heart attack, and to evaluate the heart's performance and check for heart failure. (For full description of these valuable tests, see pages 102 and 105). They may be done while you rest or exercise.

Thyroid Scan

The thyroid scan, one of the most useful types of radionuclide scanning, makes use of the fact that your thyroid needs iodine to produce its hormones. First, the doctor injects radioactive iodine into your arm vein, then he monitors the thyroid gland on a special scanner as it incorporates the radionuclide into its cells.

The test can help him to make the crucial distinction between thyroid cancers (shown by "cold areas," which do not pick up iodine) and goiters (often shown by "hot" or overactive areas). It can also aid in the diagnosis of thyroid infection and chronic inflammation ("Hashimoto's disease") as well as provide information about the gland's function.

Should a thyroid cancer be discovered and removed, injection of radioactive iodine can be used on a regular basis thereafter to scan the entire body for recurrence or spread of the cancer.

The scan is not a routine test. Physical exams and blood tests for thyroid hormone levels should precede it. However, if you develop a painful or enlarged thyroid, or symptoms of an overactive or underactive gland, it may be the only test that can provide a precise diagnosis.

Other Scans

Scans on your salivary glands may help to detect the presence of a tumor. They should be ordered whenever you have an unexplained lack of secretions in your mouth or whenever a swelling in one of the glands cannot be diagnosed by physical exam or simple x-rays.

Radionuclide scans can also be performed on your kidney and gallbladder, but in each of these cases, other techniques are proving more accurate.

ULTRASOUND

What Is the Purpose of the Test?

Ultrasound procedures are used in many different areas of the body to diagnose a wide variety of problems. They are particularly good for detecting heart disease (see page 107) and problems in the female reproductive tract (see page 126), and are used in almost 15 percent of all diagnostic imaging procedures.

How Is the Test Performed?

In all cases, a special jelly is rubbed over the area to be examined and a special transducer is passed over it. You may feel some pressure but no pain, and you will not hear or feel the sounds as the transducer bounces them off your internal organs.

Where and by Whom Should the Test Be Performed and Interpreted?

Ultrasounds can be performed by a specially trained technician in an office, hospital, or clinic. They are usually interpreted by a radiologist with experience in ultrasound interpretation.

How Accurate Is the Test?

The accuracy of ultrasound is limited in people who are very overweight, or in areas where gas or air might interfere with the image, such as in the intestine or in people with chronic lung disease. It is also difficult to perform in areas where extensive surgery has been performed, such as for heart problems in people who have had chest surgery, because scar tissue interferes with the sound waves. In most other circumstances, it is extremely accurate, and, because it carries so little risk, is sometimes the imaging procedure of choice.

What Are the Dangers of the Test?

Although some scientists speculate on the long-term effects of ultrasound tests, none has been proven and most experts consider the procedure extremely safe.

Is It Really Necessary?

Like all imaging procedures, ultrasound is rarely a first-line test and it is not on any list of routine procedures recommended for healthy people. When used properly, however, it is highly accurate and without known risk.

It may be appropriate in the following situations:

- To evaluate heart disease, especially that affecting the heart valves and heart walls (see page 107).
- To evaluate problems in the lower pelvis (see page 126) and the kidney.
- Along with nuclear scans, to evaluate testicular problems and problems of the thyroid gland.
- To follow the development of a breast cyst. In this case, ultrasound is not used to detect cancers, but may be used to observe changes in a cyst over the course of time.
- To evaluate gallbladder problems.
- To examine the prostate for early signs of cancer or to detect recurrence (see transrectal ultrasound, page 137).

Ultrasound techniques have also recently been refined to study blood vessels in a procedure called angiodynography, which produces multicolored images of the vessels as blood flows through them. The technique is being used for noninvasive study of the heart, aorta, carotid arteries, and blood vessels in the leg for blockage and other problems.

CAT OR CT (COMPUTERIZED TRANSAXIAL TOMOGRAPHY) SCANS

Imagine taking a photograph of a salami. You'd be able to see the outside surface of the salami, its shape and size and, if the picture were really clear, whether or not the surface had any irregularities. If you had a salami inside your body, that's all a simple x-ray would show you—the salami's surface.

Imagine how it would look if you could slice the salami into thin delicatessen-type slices. You'd be able to see changes inside the salami that you couldn't possibly see with the photograph. Those slices are what a CAT scan accomplishes on your internal organs.

Tomography refers to the technique of making a single x-ray picture of an isolated plane within your body, like a photo of one slice of salami without the other slices in the way to confuse the picture. The tomographic machine accomplishes this by moving as it takes the x-rays and blurring out all the other planes or slices. The CAT scan uses a computer to create clear images of the slices in each separate plane.

By using a moving x-ray machine and a computer tomography, it produces pictures of the *inside* of your organs, of "slices" at every imaginable depth and angle. It's no wonder that CAT scans have revolutionized diagnostic medicine over the past two decades. The information they yield has made seeing inside the body easier and safer while rendering other, older techniques obsolete.

What Is the Purpose of the Test?

CAT scanners were first used to diagnose brain tumors and strokes, but recent improvements have enabled them to examine virtually every area of the body. They are now used regularly to detect changes in the brain, abdomen, pelvis, chest, and back.

Their major advantage lies in their ability to study structure and anatomy; their major disadvantage in their inability to study function in an organ as it moves.

How Is the Test Performed?

During a CAT scan, you lie on a table, with the part of your body that is being studied inside a donut-shaped machine. The machine rotates around you while it shoots a tiny, precise beam of x-rays your way. In spite of the fact that numerous films are taken, the overall radiation exposure is roughly equal to that of simple x-rays, since each picture uses less radiation.

You must lie very still while the test is in progress, since the machine is programmed to isolate a certain depth within your body and blur out all others. Any movement could cause blurring of the finished picture.

Each x-ray is detected and analyzed by the computer, which then adds them all up and reproduces a cross-sectional image of each slice on a TV-type monitor. At the simple touch of a button, the technician can call up the tomogram of any depth within the organ just studied. These images remain stored within the computer and can be printed out at any time in the future.

Although their initial use was on the head, CAT scans can now be performed on almost any part of the body. They may be also be used in conjunction with dye studies to differentiate between certain problems. Under these circumstances, an initial, regular scan is taken, then dye is injected, swallowed, or given by enema, and the CAT scan is repeated.

The dyes change the appearance of some substances (such as blood) and have no effect on others such as the area within the brain that is stricken by a stroke, making precise diagnosis more possible.

Finally, CAT scans can be used in combination with radionuclide studies, such as thallium-SPECT (see page 181) to produce tomographic slices of an organ while it is working, and provide precise information about function as well as structure.

Where and by Whom Should the Test Be Performed and Interpreted?

CAT scans are usually done in the radiology department of a hospital by a radiology technician trained in the performance of CAT scans. They should be interpreted by a radiologist who has extensive experience with CAT scans, although preliminary readings may be done by an emergency or other physician who has similar training.

How Accurate Is the Test?

The accuracy of CAT scans in visualizing the structure of bone and muscle is unsurpassed by any other imaging technique. They are still the most accurate way to see certain areas of the brain, chest, and abdomen. However, their accuracy is limited when it comes to evaluating a moving organ—the motion might blur the tomographic slice. Ultrasound is superior in the study of gallbladders, for example, because gallbladders move each time you breathe, and CAT scans have been surpassed by magnetic resonance imaging (see page 177) for the study of certain organs and medical problems.

What Are the Dangers of Doing the Test?

The radiation exposure with CAT scans is similar to the exposure during a simple x-ray on the same part of your body. Brain CAT scans, for example, expose you to far less radiation than do abdominal CAT scans.

If dye studies are used in conjunction with the scan, the dangers inherent to those tests are added on, namely the possibility of allergic reaction, or of infection or bleeding at the injection site.

Is It Really Necessary?

CAT scans are rarely first-line tests. They should only be used when less complex techniques, such as simple x-rays, blood tests, and physical examination cannot produce a diagnosis. In the correct circumstances, however, CAT scans can make the difference between life and death by providing crucial information without exposing you to excessive pain or discomfort.

CAT scans should be used in the following situations:

- To diagnose unexplained headaches or nervous system disorders believed to be caused by a problem in the brain. They are excellent for the detection of brain hemorrhage due to injury, high blood pressure, or burst aneurysms. For this application, they have replaced spinal taps and have saved many lives.

  Although MRI (see below) may detect some strokes earlier than CAT scans, CAT scans are best for differentiating between a stroke and a brain hemorrhage. If the CAT scan is negative and a problem in the brain or nervous system continues, MRI studies may be indicated (see page 177).

- To detect tumors, stones, and other problems in the chest and abdomen. CAT scans not only detect tumors that simple x-rays miss, they can also define and localize the tumors that screening x-rays *do* detect.

  A CAT scan should be performed whenever a suspected tumor appears on a simple film, and whenever chest or abdominal problems are not resolved by the less complex tests. They are excellent for studying the kidney, for checking for stones and tumors, for checking the liver and pancreas for stones, tumors, and the evaluation of jaundice (yellow skin caused by excess bilirubin, see page 208), and the lungs, adrenal glands, and spleen for tumors or other growths.

- To examine the pelvis. Although ultrasound can most easily study the uterus and fallopian tubes, CAT scans are superior in other parts of the pelvis because they're not as affected by interference from bowel gas, bone, and fecal matter.

- To examine the spine for a slipped disc or tumor. CAT scans are as good or better than MRI's for the visualization of the bones and discs, but not as good for studying the spinal cord itself. Both should be considered before doing a myelogram (see page 167), which is far more dangerous than either of these imaging tests.

- To detect abnormalities in bone that fail to show up on simple x-rays.

To say that the CAT scan has helped us make major leaps in diagnostic medicine would be to understate the case. Many experts feel that it is one of the most important scientific developments of this century; even so, they have their limitations, as you can see. Discuss all of the alternatives with your doctor before deciding to have a CAT scan done.

MAGNETIC RESONANCE IMAGING (MRI)

Did you ever touch a magnet to the surface of a compass when you were a kid? If you did, you saw the needle go crazy, dancing and wobbling away from its normal position. You probably didn't realize that you were witnessing the same phenomenon that magnetic resonance imaging (MRI) depends on to see inside our bodies.

What Is the Purpose of the Test?

Like the CAT scan, MRI was first used to study the brain and nervous system, but its use has expanded far beyond that. It can be used to view the spinal cord itself, areas of the brain where CAT scans aren't clear, and many other internal organs. See below for its specific uses and for a comparison with CAT scans.

How Is the Test Performed?

We each have atoms in our body that contain an odd number of particles, called protons. When these protons are placed in a magnetic field, they wobble, much like the compass needle when you subjected it to a magnetic force.

During MRI, you are placed inside a giant cylindrical magnet, which emits a force that sends a small number of the protons in your body into a dance. They jiggle and line up, and when the pulse is turned off, they relax and return to their former position. As they return, they emit energy at a frequency that identifies them and can be detected by special radio antennas.

The frequencies are fed into a computer, which analyzes, then reconstructs them into a picture on a televisionlike monitor. The picture is precise and clear because MRI is able to detect minute differences in frequency—and it does it all without injections or radiation. As with CAT scans, dye is now being used with certain MRI tests to enhance the picture and localize medical problems in a more precise way.

Where and by Whom Should the Test Be Performed and Interpreted?

Because the magnets used in MRI are so gigantic (they may weigh as much as 100 tons), the tests are usually performed in a hospital or in a special trailer outside the hospital. They must be interpreted by a specialist who is an expert in the evaluation of MRIs.

How Accurate Are the Tests?

We are clearly in a transitional time regarding our understanding of the value of MRI's. On the one hand, many experts feel that the accuracy of MRI has been poorly studied. On the other, most of the same experts feel that it has proven to be "unusually rewarding" in the evaluation of problems of the brain, spinal cord, bones, and heart.

It appears that, like the CAT scan, MRI can detect many abnormalities that simple x-rays miss. MRI seems more accurate than CAT scans for viewing swelling, such as occurs during infections, early cancers, and early strokes. However, MRI's may not be as accurate when it comes to distinguishing between early swelling and early tumors.

They're able to view certain areas of the brain and spinal cord not clearly seen by CAT scanners. Since they can produce moving pictures, they can evaluate orthopedic problems, such as knee pain while the area is in motion, which CAT scans cannot do. Also, they can study the heart while it functions, which may eventually lead to their use as a safe, non-invasive way to study blood flow to the heart. The accuracy of MRIs in the chest, abdomen, and pelvis awaits further study, but many experts feel that they will equal or surpass CAT scanners for the study of these areas as well.

What Are the Dangers of Doing the Test?

MRI is nonradioactive, noninvasive, and believed to be harmless. There is a theoretical danger in the use of high levels of exposure to magnetic fields, but no side effects have been reported at the levels used during MRI. Long-term effects have not been studied.

The only dangers known to exist have to do with the magnet itself. MRI cannot be used on patients who have heart pacemakers, metal-containing IUD's, or metal clips on blood vessels in the brain because the magnet may cause the pacemaker to misfire, the IUD to move, or the metal clips to come loose.

Some people report feeling claustrophobic while lying inside the giant magnet and it is well known for its "projectile effect"—the ability to send unfastened metal objects soaring across the room.

Is It Really Necessary?

MRI is as much of a major step forward as was the development of CAT scans in our ability to study the inside of our bodies without invading them. Although its final place in our diagnostic tool chest is far from established, a number of things about this amazing new technology are already clear. It is painless, it appears to carry less risk than virtually all other procedures, and it is capable of providing a wide range of crucial medical information.

Its one limitation seems to be that, although it can detect differences between normal and healthy tissues, it may not be as good as some of the other tests for differentiating between types of problems. For instance, swelling from an infection may look the same as a small tumor in its early stages. For that reason, MRI must always be used along with information provided by a physical exam, symptoms, and other tests.

MRI may be appropriate in the following situations:

- To detect early brain infection, stroke, or a tumor that might be missed by a CAT scan. MRI is not as accurate for detecting brain hemorrhage, but for these other problems, it may be even more sensitive than CAT scans.
- To diagnose changes in the parts of the brain where the CAT scan is of limited use: the brain stem, the posterior area, and the area where many facial nerves exit.
- To diagnose "acoustic neuromas"—tumors of the nerve that transmits sounds from our ear to our brain.
- To diagnose multiple sclerosis, where damage is done to the protective covering of the nerves.
- To diagnose changes in joints. Because it can evaluate the joint in motion, MRI may detect tears of ligaments or structural abnormalities that regular x-rays and arthrograms might miss.

   One study showed MRI to be more accurate than bone scans for the detection of bone infections. However, because MRI is new and more expensive, it is not yet recommended as a first-line test for that diagnosis.
- To examine the spinal cord. MRI may be superior to the CAT scan for imaging the cord itself, although the CAT scan may be more precise about changes in the bones that surround it. Both tests may precede the more dangerous myelogram (see page 167).
- To study the heart. This is one of the newer uses of MRI, and its

value here is still being tested. Recent studies have shown that it may be as accurate as the CAT scan and angiography for checking to see whether the coronary arteries remain unblocked after coronary artery bypass surgery. MRI may one day make safe, "noninvasive" angiography possible.

● The use of MRI in the diagnosis of other problems is still being reviewed. One researcher is even studying its ability to detect changes in the brain during what has been labeled "chronic fatigue syndrome" (see page 205).

MRI clearly has great potential. Its eventual use may range from simple tests on joints to life-saving tests that can evaluate the condition of the arteries that bring blood to the heart. For the present, though, its use is limited by the size of the magnet, its cost (which is higher than most other imaging tests), and the fact that its overall accuracy is still being tested.

Positron Emission Tomography (PET Scan)

Positron emission tomography—a combination CAT and radionuclide scan—does more than allow us to see the anatomy of an organ; it allows us to study its performance as well.

The doctor injects a radionuclide that has been chemically attached to a normal biological substance such as sugar into your body. As this substance travels through your body, it emits positrons—which are faster moving and higher in energy than the particles emitted during other nuclear scans. Special detectors pick up the energy and feed it into a computer, which then translates it into a multicolored picture on a special monitor. Since your organs are scanned as they use the substance, the PET test provides unique functional information about each organ's health and is capable of detecting very early signs of disease.

PET scanners are rare (there are fewer than twenty in the United States) and expensive, but experts feel that they will take us another major step forward in our ability to examine and evaluate the health of our internal organs.

The PET scan is already being used for the following purposes:

● To study the brain and determine if coma is irreversible
● To evaluate depression
● To study the nature of cancer and follow the response of tumors to treatment
● To diagnose heart disease while it is still reversible

Thallium Single Photon Emission Computerized Tomography (SPECT)

SPECT is a scanning procedure that also combines some of the features of radionuclide and CAT scans (see page 173).

In one of its most common uses, the radionuclide thallium is injected into an arm vein and taken up by normal heart cells that have adequate blood flow. These areas are seen as "hot spots" on the scanner. Cells that have died because of a heart attack or that are not receiving enough blood appear as "cold spots."

If your doctor were to review the test at this point, as is done after a simple thallium heart scan (see page 102, he'd be able to tell whether your heart was getting enough blood, and infer whether or not a coronary artery was blocked. By doing a SPECT test with the addition of a CAT-type scanner, he can get even more information. Since this scanner will provide him with visual "slice" views of what the thallium does at every depth *inside* the heart, he'll be able to tell exactly where an abnormality begins and where it ends. He'll know more about whether the problem is reversible and how to plan a course of treatment.

Currently, thallium-SPECT scans of the heart are available only at major universities, but their use, as well as that of SPECT scans on other parts of the body, is sure to become more widespread over the course of the next few years.

THE IMAGING TECHNIQUES: A COMPARISON

Simple X-rays

ADVANTAGES
1. Least expensive.
2. Takes just a few minutes for tests and results.

DISADVANTAGES
1. Radiation exposure.
2. Limited view. Flat and two-dimensional, may miss some abnormalities.

Dye Studies

ADVANTAGES
1. More detailed view of inside of hollow organs.

DISADVANTAGES
1. Risks of injection (bleeding or infection) or allergic reaction.
2. Equal or greater exposure to radiation.

Nuclear Scans

ADVANTAGES
1. More detail of the anatomy of certain organs.
2. Ability to study organ in motion, while it functions.
3. Possibly less overall radiation than with x-rays.
4. Some are portable and can be brought to the bedside.

DISADVANTAGES
1. Risk of injection as above, and of allergic reaction.
2. More radiation than with MRI.
3. Certain areas of body not well visualized with scans.

Ultrasound (see pelvic, page 126, and heart, page 107)

ADVANTAGES
1. Although theoretical risk exists, none has been demonstrated.
2. No injections, dyes, or radiation necessary.
3. Least expensive of the newer techniques.
4. May be portable—brought to bedside.
5. Good for differentiating fluid from solids.

DISADVANTAGES
1. Very limited in obese patients. May be unable to diagnose up to 20 percent of patients for this reason.
2. Is blocked by bowel gas or bone, therefore is less diagnostically useful on many different body parts.

CAT Scans

ADVANTAGES
1. Clear "slice" views of the inner body at successive depths. Provides details of inside of organs. As a consequence, will pick up many things that simple x-rays miss while not increasing the dangers.
2. Excellent on bone and muscle.
3. Excellent for detecting brain hemorrhage.
4. Can use dye to distinguish between brain hemorrhage and stroke.

DISADVANTAGES
1. Risk of radiation near or equal to that of simple x-rays.
2. Cannot image moving areas as well as MRI.
3. Less accurate than other tests in imaging certain parts of the brain (brain stem, for instance) and spinal cord.

MRI

ADVANTAGES
1. No known risk; studies of long-term risk have not been done.
2. No injections.
3. Capable of imaging moving areas.
4. Can image at any angle, more so than CAT scanners.
5. Can detect swelling earlier than CAT scan; may pick up infection or stroke earlier.

DISADVANTAGES
1. Currently the most expensive imaging test.
2. Cannot be used on patients with heart pacemakers, metal-containing IUD's or metal clips on blood vessels in the brain.
3. Many patients feel very claustrophobic within the magnet.
4. Although detects swelling earlier, may not be able to distinguish from other problems.

PET Scans

ADVANTAGES
1. Can study function and metabolism as well as structure.

DISADVANTAGES
1. New technique and few PET scanners are available.

SPECT

ADVANTAGE
1. Can determine exact area of abnormality.

DISADVANTAGES
1. Tomography must be done while lying still, therefore not as efficient for exercise studies.

HOW TO DECIDE WHICH, IF ANY, IMAGING TEST
YOU NEED

1. If your doctor suggests such a test, discuss the advantages and disadvantages of that test with him.
2. Consider whether you have any contraindications to that test. If you wear a heart pacemaker, for instance, you may not be able to take an MRI.
3. Consider the cost, and the risks of the test, and weigh those against the need for it—what it may reveal and whether or not the results will affect your treatment. A test which cannot provide information that might alter treatment rarely needs to be done.
4. Read the more detailed description of the test in this chapter.
5. Discuss the alternatives with your doctor.

In considering which is the best imaging test for each body area or each type of problem, you need to remember that they are rarely first-line tests. Often, other, simpler, tests should precede them in order to narrow down the diagnosis and let you know exactly what the imaging test will be searching for.

WHICH TEST IS RIGHT FOR WHICH PROBLEM?

Bone Infection

Although one recent study suggested that the MRI might be most accurate, the nuclear bone scan is still the gold standard. This may change in the next few years.

Bone Fractures, Tumors, and Joint Problems

Simple x-rays should be the first-line test, followed by a CAT scan for fractures that might be missed on a simple x-ray (especially those in facial bones, which infrequently require a CAT scan), and by MRI for detecting subtle changes in cartilage, tendons, and ligaments while the joint moves. Arthogram may be useful in joint problems as well, but it's more invasive and risky than either of the other two.

Brain and Nervous System Problems

MRI is better than the CAT scan where bone interferes: in the brain stem, cerebellum, and posterior area. In all other cases, the following are considered the imaging tests of choice for the detection of the specific problem.

Hemorrhage and injury   CAT scans are the best test.

Aneurysms   Angiogram is the definitive test, followed by MRI in accuracy. CAT scans may be used if the aneurysms burst and bleed.

Stroke   MRI may detect strokes earlier, but CAT scans are best for distinguishing between stroke and hemorrhage.

Infection and swelling   MRI may detect these earlier than CAT scans.

Hydrocephalus (water on the brain)   MRI is more sensitive than CAT scans.

Demylinating diseases like multiple sclerosis.   MRI is currently the only imaging test used to aid in the diagnosis of these diseases.

Acoustic neuromas   MRI is clearly superior to other imaging tests for the detection of these tumors of the "hearing" nerve.

Spine

Spinal bones   CAT scans are slightly superior to MRI.

Spinal cord   MRI is superior.

Both tests should probably be preceded by simple x-ray and may, in turn, precede the more dangerous myelogram.

Chest

Tumors and infections   In the chest, screen for these conditions by using simple x-rays, followed by a CAT scan if the diagnosis is unclear. The CAT scan is excellent in the mediastinum—the midchest area where simple x-rays yield poor results.

The heart   Radionuclide scanning is most precise for evaluating function and endangered areas; angiography is most specific for coronary artery disease; and ultrasound is best for problems with the heart valves. Radionuclide scanning with CAT scans (SPECT) shows great promise, as does MRI of the heart.

The lungs   Simple x-rays are still the best screening test, although the CAT scan is used for more precise definition of tumors and other problems. The lung scan is the most useful noninvasive test for pulmonary embolism.

Breast

Mammography is clearly the imaging test of choice.

Abdomen

Gallbladder   For detecting infection, nuclear scans are replacing ultrasound tests in many institutions.

For gallstones, ultrasound may be best, after a simple x-ray has been taken to screen for their presence.

Liver and spleen   Radionuclide scans and CAT scans are both used to diagnose tumors and other problems.

Pancreas   CAT scans are considered superior to other imaging tests for evaluation of the pancreas, although an older, more invasive test called ERCP (Endoscopic retrograde cholangio-pancreatogram) (a study involving the injection of dye into the pancreatic area) may be as accurate.

Kidney   For infection and kidney stones, a simple x-ray should be performed first, followed, if necessary, by dye studies.

For tumors and injury and to a lesser extent stones, CAT scans may be employed.

Preliminary reports suggest that MRI may be as accurate as CAT scans in detecting a change in the kidney (seeing the first signs of swelling or tumor) but not in making a precise diagnosis.

The Pelvis and Genital Areas

Scrotum   Nuclear scans and ultrasound are best for the evaluation of sudden, severe pain or growths.

Lower female pelvis   Ultrasound is best; used to detect tubal pregnancies, infections, and other problems.

Pelvis   Above the pubic bones, CAT scans are superior.

Prostate   Ultrasound is proving accurate and useful for detecting prostate cancer; CAT scans and MRI's are still being studied.

Hollow Organs: Blood Vessels, Stomach, Intestine, and Esophagus

Endoscopic exams combined with dye studies seem to be the most accurate, although they are invasive and should be used only when symptoms, history, or other findings suggest that they are needed.

CAT scans can detect some abnormalities, and MRI is being investigated for use in these areas.

All of these imaging techniques have helped to change the face of medicine. Many scientists believe that the time is coming when you'll be able to walk into a booth and have all of your blood chemistries and internal organs checked out without experiencing any discomfort or danger—and without seeing the doctor. If that ever happens, you won't have to choose from among different imaging tests, but you'll really have to know how to interpret results. With all the options now, while you don't need interpretation skills, you do have to know how to choose.

A recent report in the *Journal of the American Medical Association* claimed that for nearly 20 percent of patients who underwent costly, somewhat dangerous, angiography of the heart, the test was unnecessary. If your doctor suggests that you undergo one of these imaging techniques, discuss it with him at length—and don't be afraid to ask questions or consider alternatives. Read the description of the test here and consider its purpose, advantages, disadvantages, and risks before deciding to have it done. You'll be protecting both your pocketbook and your health.

FOURTEEN

Tests on Your Urine and Blood

Your body is made up of nearly 60 percent water, two-thirds of it within your cells and one third in body compartments and blood vessels.

Each day you exchange some of this fluid with your environment. Fluids carry waste out of your body and nutrients in; fluids protect you against disease and transport hormones to your internal organs where they can work to keep you healthy.

The testing of this fluid is the simplest of all medical tests. With a simple container for urine and a needle and syringe for blood and other bodily fluids, your doctor can obtain all sorts of diagnostic information. Perhaps for this reason, many body fluid tests are performed too frequently in today's fitness-conscious, prevention-minded world.

You may see signs at your health club for a "complete preventive checkup, including blood and urine tests to screen for illness and risk of disease," or receive a soliciting piece of mail or phone call offering the same sort of opportunity. Unfortunately, you may only learn later on that your insurance doesn't cover you for preventive tests or that they were run at the wrong times, under the wrong circumstances. For instance, a blood cholesterol level drawn in the middle of the day after a heavy meal may not reflect your true cholesterol level. Your doctor may be unable to interpret it and you won't know what to do about it.

The only way to ensure that tests on your bodily fluids produce accurate, fruitful information is to learn which are necessary for you, and when and how each should be performed.

Review the blood and urine tests that are considered routine for your age group in Chapter Six, then read their description here to make sure you prepare properly for them, and that they're interpreted correctly. Whenever a new or different test is suggested, review its description here and consider your medical needs before having it done.

TESTS ON YOUR URINE

Your urine is the result of a long bodily process. Blood that reaches the kidney has already passed through every other organ and has been used to carry nutrients, assist metabolic functions, and deliver energy where needed. The kidney completes the process by filtering the fluid, making sure you hold on to minerals and other substances you need and excrete those you don't need, or that could harm you. The finished product, your urine, can provide information about the health of each of these organs as well as about the kidney itself.

What Is the Purpose of Urine Tests?

By running one or more of the almost one hundred urine lab tests that now exist, your doctor can learn a great deal about your health. Urine tests can provide information about infections, hormonal imbalances, drug use, diabetes, kidney, liver or heart problems, and a whole host of other illnesses.

How Are Urine Tests Performed?

You will usually be asked to collect the urine sample yourself. You will be given a sterile plastic or glass container and instructed as to its use. For most tests, you need to void about a quarter cup of urine into the container. In many cases, the sample needs to be taken to the lab within an hour, or else covered securely and refrigerated until it can be brought there. For certain tests, the sample must be obtained at a certain time of the day—in the case of a pregnancy test, for instance, the first thing in the morning. Other tests require that the sample be produced only after taking foods or medications.

Urine tests that check for signs of infection must be done very carefully: first the genital area must be cleaned with swabs and antiseptic, then urine must be collected from the middle of the flow (not the first few drops of flow) in a special sterile container obtained from the doctor. If your doctor asks for this kind of sample (it's known as a "clean-catch midstream specimen"), make sure to follow the instructions precisely.

At one time or another you may also be asked to collect all your urine over a twenty-four-hour period (a "timed specimen"). In those circumstances, you will need to be careful to collect *all* your urine during that time, and you will need to keep the sample refrigerated throughout the day.

Lastly, in cases where the kidney or bladder is obstructed, it may be necessary for the urine to be obtained via a thin rubber tube ("catheter") inserted through the urethra (the tube that brings urine from your bladder to the outside) into the bladder. When the urethra is blocked or diseased, a needle may have to be employed to collect the urine through a tiny puncture in your lower abdomen.

Whatever the method of collection, though, it is important for you to remember that urine that has been collected improperly or stored incorrectly can seriously affect the accuracy of your test results.

Where Should the Sample Be Taken, Who Should Collect It, and Who Should Interpret the Results?

A lab technician can tell you what kind of urine sample is called for in your case, and you can usually collect it yourself at home. You should consult with your doctor about the procedure if he asks you to take a twenty-four-hour "timed sample."

A nurse or doctor will need to make the collection if a catheter is required, and a doctor should draw the urine if a needle is used. In both of these cases, the sample can be taken in the doctor's office, at your home if your doctor is making a house-call, or in a clinic or hospital.

How Accurate Are Urine Tests?

Tests on urine samples for infection and urine analysis (see below) are generally very accurate, if you follow the collection instructions carefully.

Tests to identify specific minerals and other substances in the urine are more difficult, but are likely to be accurate if the test is performed and the results evaluated correctly.

What Are the Dangers Involved in Urine Tests?

No danger is involved in the regular collection of urine, except if the results are misinterpreted for some reason.

When the sample is obtained using a catheter or needle, there is about a 2 to 3 percent risk of bladder infection. This can be minimized by making sure the urine is taken with thorough, sterile technique: sterile gloves should be worn, and the area should be cleaned with antiseptic before the sample is collected.

Are Urine Tests Really Necessary?

Some urine tests are certainly appropriate and may even be necessary. Others are not necessary, and some are done too frequently or at inappropriate times.

Routine Urine Analysis

A routine or "complete" urine analysis consists of a number of the most common urine tests, all performed at the same time on one sample. It is one of the most reliable screening tests, and is often routinely administered in conjunction with a general medical checkup. It can provide your doctor with information about bladder infection, blood disease, liver disease, urinary tract problems, diabetes, kidney stones, hormone disorders, high blood pressure, and many other problems.

A urine analysis will usually include tests for the volume, color, specific gravity (a measure of how concentrated the urine is), and acidity (pH) of the urine, as well as for the presence in the urine of bacteria, blood cells, crystals, proteins, sugar, or debris.

A twenty-four-hour urine analysis may be necessary to check the overall volume of urine, or to investigate the total amounts of the various substances listed above that are excreted in a day, as well as to check for other problems such as hormonal disturbances and gout (the uric acid level is the relevant test in this case).

Children should have a urine analysis once in the first year of life, once at age 4, once between the ages of 6 and 11, and once between 12 and 17.

Adults should be tested routinely once between ages 18 and 25, then at five-year intervals until age 60, every 2½ years between 60 and 75, and once a year thereafter.

You will also require a urine analysis anytime you develop urinary symptoms.

Urine Tests for Sugar

There is normally no detectable amount of sugar, or glucose, in the urine, so the presence of sugar may indicate the presence of a disease such as diabetes.

Urine tests for sugar are done routinely at the time of urine analysis, but the separate, more precise test should only be performed if you find yourself experiencing the common symptoms of diabetes such as excessive thirst and urination.

Urine Tests for Infection

Bladder infections are very common in women and rare in men, because the woman's urethra is shorter than the man's and also closer to the anus, the source of many of the bacteria that can cause these infections. Also, although both men and women can suffer from kidney infections, women do so more frequently.

Urine is tested for infection only when symptoms appear, such as frequency or pain on urination, discharge from the urethra (which could indicate an STD—see page 211), blood in the urine, or back pain and fever (signs of kidney infection). In these cases, the urine samples should be a sterile "clean-catch midstream specimen." If the results of the tests are negative, but the symptoms warrant further analysis, the test may have to be repeated, and a culture may have to be taken.

Since men are not routinely prone to urinary infections, a positive test in a man should lead to further workup. It may first be necessary to rule out the possibility of prostatitis, or infection of the prostate, by collecting sterile urine samples before and after rectal exam and prostate massage (see also page 55). If prostatitis is not the cause, an IVP and/or a cystoscopy (see pages 167 and 148) may be necessary to determine the cause of the infection.

NOTE: If you have a urinary discharge—whitish or yellowish fluid coming from your urethra—or you've been exposed to a sexually transmitted disease (STD), even if you don't have any symptoms special tests may need to be run on your blood and/or urine, as well as on the discharge. See the chapter on tests for STD's, page 211.

Urine Tests for the Presence of Blood

The test for blood in the urine may be performed as a routine portion of your urine analysis. If it is discovered during that test, if you notice obvious blood in your urine (even if you feel no pain), or if your urine becomes darker, the more specific test may need to be performed. Although dark urine may be caused by eating beets, blackberries, food coloring, B complex vitamins, or any of a dozen laxatives and other drugs, you shouldn't take a chance by omitting a urine test.

When blood *is* found in your urine, it could mean you have kidney disease or some other problem in the urinary tract that needs attending to.

Urine Tests for Crystals

Most urine analyses include a microscopic analysis of the sediment in the urine, but they may or may not routinely detect the presence of crystals in the urine. Under certain circumstances, special microscopes with special types of light may be the only way to find the crystals.

The test may be done if you develop kidney stones, gout, or other problems your doctor believes are due to crystal deposits in your body. In these cases, you may also need a blood test to measure your blood uric acid level (see page 203), and in the case of gout, the affected joint may need to be tapped (see page 154) to look for crystals.

Other Urine Tests

Urine can also be evaluated for the presence of following:

- The presence and exact levels of your hormones.
- Bilirubin, a by-product of the breakdown of red blood cells whose presence may suggest the presence of blood or liver disease.
- Protein, which may suggest kidney disease.
- Various vitamins and minerals.
- Electrolytes such as sodium, potassium, and carbon dioxide, which may yield information about the health of your kidneys, lungs, and other organs.
- Drugs and medicines, to determine whether poisoning or illegal drug use has occurred, or to measure the level of prescription medicines and make sure they are in the desired range. This test may also be performed on your blood.

TESTS ON YOUR BLOOD

Your blood is made up of about 50 percent cells and 50 percent fluid. Red blood cells (RBC's) carry oxygen to your cells and organs, white blood cells (WBC's) fight infection, and the tiny cells called platelets help the blood to clot. The fluid contains vitamins, hormones, nutrients, and other chemicals.

What Is the Purpose of These Tests?

Blood samples are taken to test for the presence of abnormal substances in the blood, to pick up higher or lower than normal levels of substances that are normally present, and to pick up changes in your blood's overall makeup.

How Are Blood Tests Performed?

The simplest way to draw a blood sample is by a pinprick on your finger or thumb. Larger samples are usually obtained from the veins, often at your elbow, using a needle and syringe. Samples of arterial blood can also be collected using a syringe, but this test is usually performed at the wrist or groin area, and it may be more painful than the other two tests.

Where and by Whom Should the Test Be Performed and Interpreted?

Blood samples can be drawn at home, in the doctor's office, or at a hospital or clinic. A technician can draw the sample, and an appropriate specialist such as your doctor or a pathologist should evaluate the results.

Are the Tests Accurate?

The accuracy of blood tests depends on what the blood is being tested for, on the technician performing the test, and on the doctor who interprets it.

Blood-cell counts are usually extremely accurate, but some of the newer tests, such as those used for the identification of antibodies, hormones, or oncofetal antigens (see page 206) have not been studied for as long, and their interpretation and use may be subject to more question.

What Are the Dangers of Doing These Tests?

There is very little risk involved in taking a blood test, although you may experience some mild bruising at the place where the blood was drawn. More serious but rare complications include the formation of blood clots, infection at the site where the blood was drawn, and infection of the circulating blood.

Are These Tests Really Necessary?

Many blood tests are routine. Some are necessary only occasionally. Others are used far too frequently or inappropriately.

Review the blood tests considered routine for your age group in Chapter Six, then read their description here to make sure that you prepare properly for them and that they're interpreted correctly. Whenever a new or different test is suggested, review its description here and consider your own medical needs before having it done.

THE ROUTINE BLOOD TESTS

The only blood tests that should be recommended on a routine basis for healthy people are those for hemoglobin and hematocrit, blood lipids and blood sugar. Nevertheless, some tests, called "packages" or "panels," are ordered every time you visit the doctor. Each of these packages includes a number of tests offered at a lower price than they would cost if each were paid for individually. While each has its value when ordered appropriately, you should check with your doctor before having them done. Make sure you really need all the items in the group, and that the total cost of the group is less than the cost of the individual tests you need, or you may find yourself paying for unnecessary tests.

Complete Blood Count (CBC)

The CBC is the most commonly performed lab test. Blood is drawn by a technician or a doctor, then analyzed under a microscope by a technician. The test measures your hemoglobin and hematocrit, your red blood cell count, white blood cell count, and platelet count.

Hemoglobin is a protein found within the red blood cells. It holds the oxygen as it's carried from the lungs to the body's tissues.

Hematocrit is a measure of what percentage of your blood is made up of red blood cells.

The hemoglobin and hematocrit are the only tests that are recommended on a routine basis, being suggested twice in the first five years of life, then once during each of the separate life periods listed in the table beginning on page 286.

Both numbers may drop as a result of bleeding, iron deficiency, kidney disease, and a whole variety of other disorders. In addition to routine testing, they may need to be rechecked in the following circumstances:

● If your doctor is concerned because you show signs of possible blood loss
● After an injury or before and after an operation
● If you have a suspected ulcer, blood in your stool, or feel unusually weak and light-headed
● If your skin has turned paler than is usual for you

The *red blood cell count* can tell your doctor if you have too few red blood cells (which can also occur as a result of bleeding or other problems), or too many. Too many RBC's is a condition called polycythemia, which may make you feel weak and lethargic, and usually needs treatment.

RBC counts are not done routinely but may be indicated if any of these symptoms occur.

The *white blood cell count* increases in response to pain, stress, inflammation, or infection, especially in bacterial infections; in viral infections, the total count may drop.

Since there are a number of different types of white cells, this count and examination can also tell doctors about the possibility of such different problems as allergic reaction or leukemia, and about the body's response to chemotherapy in the treatment of cancer.

Platelets are the tiny, cell fragments that play a role in blood clotting. A platelet count is usually included in a routine CBC. A platelet count should be ordered, along with the clotting tests listed on page 199, whenever you have any sign of easy bruising, or abnormal or prolonged clotting times.

Blood Lipids

Almost 30 percent of the nearly 2 million deaths in this country each year are the result of coronary artery disease (CAD), the risk of which we know to be increased by elevated levels of blood cholesterol. For this reason, lipid testing has become a routine blood test, but many people are confused about which lipids should be checked for, and when. In order to understand the different tests, and what you need to do about the various results, you must understand how your body handles fat.

When we eat a fatty meal, the fat is broken down into cholesterol and other substances, then absorbed into the blood and carried throughout the body by various lipoproteins, which are complexes consisting of a fat and a protein.

High-density lipoproteins (HDL's) are believed to take cholesterol to the liver, where it can be removed from the body without causing harm.

Low-density lipoproteins (LDL's) take cholesterol to blood vessels, where it may cause blockage and lead to coronary artery disease.

HDL's are therefore thought to be good for you, and LDL's to be bad.

THE CHOLESTEROL COUNT   When it comes to measuring risk of heart disease due to blood lipids, your total blood cholesterol count is still the most important number. The National Cholesterol Education Program guidelines urge all Americans over 20 to have their blood cholesterol tested, and suggests that further tests should be made at least every five years.

What do the figures mean? The number expresses mg/dl, milligrams per decaliter.

Under 200   Desirable.

200–219   Borderline; slight increased risk. Consider lowering your cholesterol with dietary restrictions.

220–239   Moderate to high risk. Dietary restriction should be undertaken. Medicine may be necessary if there are other risk factors, such as high blood pressure, obesity, cigarette smoking or diabetes.

Over 240   High risk. Take aggressive steps to reduce with diet; medicine may be required as well.

Over 300   Probable lipid disease. Take immediate steps with your doctor to evaluate the problem and determine which therapy is needed. In the past, this was the cut-off number before any treatment—even dietary—was begun. We've since learned better.

LOW-DENSITY LIPOPROTEINS (LDL'S)   LDL is now considered a risk factor.

Less than 130   Desirable.

130–159   Borderline to high. Consider dietary therapy. Medicine may be necessary if you have other risk factors such as high blood pressure or obesity, or you smoke cigarettes or have diabetes.

More than 160   High risk. Consider medical treatment.

More than 190   Medical treatment is essential.

HIGH-DENSITY LIPOPROTEINS (HDL'S)   Although many experts believe that your blood HDL level is significant, long-term studies on the ability of HDL's to reduce health risks haven't been completed. For the time being, therefore, the major lipid risk factors are considered to be total cholesterol and LDL levels.

This actually takes the HDL into account anyway, since the HDL level is included in your total cholesterol count. Total cholesterol minus your LDL gives a rough approximation of your HDL. Therefore, a cholesterol count of 230 with an HDL count of 50 may be safer than a cholesterol count of 225 with an HDL of 30.

All of these numbers should be taken into account when you are planning your approach to the measurement and control of your blood lipids.

If diabetes or other risk factors exist, or if your doctor suspects a lipid disease, a condition where your body processes fat poorly, you may want to measure your triglyceride level as well. You should know, however, that triglyceride levels by themselves have not proved to be a consistent risk factor in the development of coronary artery disease.

YOUR DIET AND YOUR BLOOD LIPID LEVELS   Although one in five hundred people has an inherited tendency to have very high blood cholesterol levels, most people can lower their blood cholesterol levels by following a lower-fat, lower-cholesterol diet. Studies suggest that a program of this kind can usually achieve a 10 to 15 percent reduction in blood cholesterol. The benefits of lowering your cholesterol level are very real: for every point that a high or moderate cholesterol level goes down, there is a 2 percent decrease in the risk of heart disease.

TESTS FOR BLOOD SUGAR

Blood sugar tests are performed by the doctor to diagnose diabetes or hypoglycemia (low blood sugar), or may be done in the home by the diabetic who has been instructed how to monitor the effects of his treatment. Blood sugar tests are suggested as routine screening tests once between the ages of 25 and 39, once every five years until age 60, every two years between 60 and 75, and every year thereafter. You may also be checked if you exhibit symptoms of low blood sugar, such as light-headedness or unexplained losses of consciousness, or of high blood sugar and diabetes, such as excessive thirst and urination.

Blood sugar tests are most accurate when performed early in the morning, after a twelve- or fourteen-hour fast. If the initial reading leads your doctor to suspect diabetes, the level may be checked more often in order to guide treatment.

A *glucose tolerance test* is more precise for determining the cause of high or low blood sugar than are simple blood sugar tests. The test involves eating a high-carbohydrate diet for several days, then drinking a special concentrated sugar solution. The doctor or technician will measure the blood glucose level at regular intervals over the next several hours to determine how the body handles a sugar load.

Glucose tolerance tests are normally performed at a hospital or clinic and are indicated only when a diagnosis of high or low blood sugar cannot be made with a simple blood test.

ENZYME AND HORMONAL TESTS IN THE NEWBORN BABY

These tests check for thyroid disease and diseases such as phenylketonuria and galactosemia, which are both inherited metabolic disorders.

Your obstetrician or pediatrician may order them routinely for your baby immediately after birth, and may repeat them at a later date if they turn out to be abnormal. Many thyroid and genetic problems are treatable if caught early enough.

TESTS FOR BLOOD TYPE

These tests determine the type (A, B, AB, or O) and subtype (Rh positive or Rh negative) of your blood, by measuring certain markers and antibodies in your blood. Since they tell us which bloods are compatible, they are appropriate in three specific situations:

- At an early age, so that you will always know your blood type, should you ever need or want to give a blood transfusion. This type stays the same throughout your lifetime.
- If you don't know your type, both your blood and that of the prospective donor or recipient should be tested when you are about to give or receive a blood transfusion. Mixing incompatible blood types can be fatal.
- During your first pregnancy, since an Rh-negative mother who has an Rh-positive child needs to be injected with a specific immunoglobulin immediately after delivery.

  This will prevent the mother's blood from forming antibodies that might attack the blood of any future Rh-positive babies, a consequence that could cause injury or death to the baby.

TESTS FOR CLOTTING TIME

There are many different ways to test the clotting time of blood. These include prothrombin time, partial thromboplastin time, and ivy bleeding time.

The tests are not routine, and should only be ordered under the following circumstances:

- Whenever you experience prolonged (more than a few minutes) or abnormal bleeding.
- Whenever you are taking "blood thinners." These medicines purposely prolong bleeding times to prevent clots from forming on arti-

ficial heart valves, or to treat "thrombophlebitis," which is inflammation and clots in the leg veins. In these circumstances, the tests are done to make sure the dose is in the desired range and not excessive.

- Whenever your doctor suspects that you have a bleeding disorder like hemophilia. If his suspicions are confirmed, he may order tests for levels of specific clotting factors.

TESTS FOR BLOOD IRON

The iron contained in red blood cells helps the cell to hold on to oxygen. If your iron level is low, your blood's ability to bring oxygen to your tissues is reduced.

Bodily iron can be reduced by a number of problems, including blood loss, chronic inflammation, or iron deficiency due to dietary or stomach and intestinal problems.

A simple measurement of your blood iron level may or may not lead to a clear diagnosis or a definitive treatment. Therefore, if your doctor suspects that you are low in iron, he may decide to measure both your iron and iron-binding levels. The combination of these two tests with your red blood cell count, hemoglobin, and hematocrit levels will enable him to decide whether or not you need treatment. If you do, he will know whether it should consist of diet, iron medication, or blood transfusion.

CALCIUM, PHOSPHORUS, AND MAGNESIUM

The testing of your blood for these mineral levels is not routine. A well-balanced, normal diet should provide all the minerals and vitamins you need, and the level of calcium in a postmenopausal woman's blood is not a good measure of whether or not she needs calcium supplements. Since bone changes that occur in osteoporosis may not cause a change in blood calcium levels. However, because certain conditions can cause dangerously high or low levels of calcium and other minerals, there are circumstances under which it's appropriate to measure your blood levels:

- When symptoms such as tiredness, muscle twitching, weakness, or abnormal heart rhythms lead your doctor to suspect abnormally low or high levels of these minerals
- To evaluate cancer or bone problems, kidney disease, or disease of the parathyroid gland, all of which can affect your blood levels of these important minerals
- When your doctor suspects a deficiency in vitamin D, which should lead him to check phosphorus and calcium levels in a test for para-

thyroid disease, or folic acid (such as occurs in people who abuse alcohol and turn out to have low levels of magnesium)

YOUR BLOOD ELECTROLYTES: SODIUM, POTASSIUM, CHLORIDE, AND BICARBONATE

Tests for these elements may be ordered as part of a panel of tests that includes blood sugar, BUN and creatinine (see next page) or each can be ordered separately. None of the tests is specifically recommended as a part of your infrequent routine checkups. Make sure they are not ordered routinely unless there are specific indications for them, such as:

● Whenever the doctor suspects an electrolyte problem
● If you have a history of such problems
● If you have a history of kidney, heart, or liver disease or diabetes, all of which can lead to electrolyte disturbances and need to be followed routinely
● If you develop symptoms of electrolyte problems such as water retention, weakness, or lethargy
● If you have symptoms that could lead to electrolyte problems such as vomiting, diarrhea, or dehydration
● If you take diuretics or "water pills," which may cause the loss of some electrolytes, especially potassium

BLOOD CARBON DIOXIDE (CO_2)

The amount of carbon dioxide carried in your blood can be affected by a wide variety of disorders, including lung, liver, and kidney problems. The test may be specifically called for in cases of suspected heart failure, hyperventilation, lung or kidney problems, or diabetes.

CO_2 can be measured in blood taken from your vein, by calculating it from the blood bicarbonate level, or directly, by measuring CO_2 as an arterial blood gas (see page 202).

CARBON MONOXIDE (CO)

Carbon monoxide is not a normal constituent of blood. It can, however, reach the blood if it is breathed in from automobile fumes, fires, home heaters, and certain industrial locations.

Carbon monoxide can kill you quickly by crippling the action of hemoglobin etc., or build up in your blood over time.

The amount in your bloodstream is measured by testing for carboxyhemoglobin, an end product of CO's interaction with hemoglobin. The test should be run whenever carbon monoxide poisoning is suspected, or whenever you've been exposed to any of the above sources and develop breathing difficulty, weakness, or disorientation.

BLOOD UREA NITROGEN (BUN)

Blood urea is the end result of protein metabolism in the body. It's found in the blood in the form of blood urea nitrogen (BUN). Blood urea levels may become higher when there are kidney, liver, or blood problems, and lower in cases of excessive fluid intake, liver disease, and malnutrition. A BUN test may be part of a "package" for blood chemistries test, or may be ordered in conjunction with any of the problems listed above.

BLOOD CREATININE

One way to evaluate the health of your kidneys is to measure how effective they are at filtering and excreting creatinine, one of the waste products of muscle metabolism. If your blood levels go up, it means that the kidney is not filtering as much creatinine as it should. The levels can also go up as a result of muscle problems, but healthy kidneys should be able to excrete the excess amount. In most cases, an elevated blood creatinine is a sign of kidney failure.

Your doctor may measure your creatinine if he suspects kidney disease or if you develop symptoms consistent with kidney problems, such as unexplained anemia, weakness, or changes in your body fluid and electrolyte balance. Diabetics, who are at increased risk for developing kidney problems, may need to have their creatinine checked on a regular basis.

In either case, if your creatinine is high, the doctor may suggest a twenty-four-hour testing of your urine and blood for a creatinine clearance evaluation, which will provide a more precise measure of kidney function.

ARTERIAL BLOOD GASES

The test for blood gases measures the pH (acidity and/or alkalinity) of the blood, and the amount of oxygen and carbon dioxide dissolved in it.

It's performed by taking blood from an artery (usually in your wrist or groin) rather than a vein, which is the source of most other blood samples. This procedure is slightly painful and slightly more dangerous than other blood tests, since arteries are actively pumping blood. You may want to ask for some local numbing medicine before the test and make sure that someone applies pressure to the spot where the needle went in for a full five minutes after the test, to prevent bleeding.

Blood gas tests may be ordered to determine the pH factor and oxygen and carbon dioxide levels in the following circumstances:

- Heart attack and/or heart failure
- Chronic or acute lung disease
- Severe diabetic complications that lead to coma
- Severe or acute kidney or liver disease
- Hyperventilation or difficulty breathing
- Drug overdose

In all of these cases, the results should help the doctor narrow down the cause of the problem and decide whether additional oxygen or other forms of treatment are needed.

BLOOD HORMONAL LEVELS

These tests measure the levels of your body's various hormones: thyroid, adrenal, pituitary, testosterone, estrogen, and progesterone among them. Blood hormone tests are not routine, but your doctor may order one if he suspects that a problem exists in one of your hormone-secreting glands.

If the results are abnormal, he may then suggest a hormonal stimulation test. Such a test involves the injection of a medication that causes your body either to increase or decrease its output of a certain hormone, which helps your doctor diagnose the exact cause of the abnormality. Since they are more dangerous than the simple hormone tests, they should only be performed and interpreted by an expert, such as an internist who has been trained in the diagnosis of hormonal disorders.

BLOOD URIC ACID

Uric acid is one of the by-products of the natural breakdown of the body's cells. Some people make too much uric acid, or their bodies do not excrete enough of it. Certain treatments, such as chemotherapy for leukemia, increase the breakdown rate of cells, and thus the production of uric acid. In all three cases, the extra uric acid may collect in joints to produce gout or in kidneys to produce kidney stones.

Blood uric acid level is not a routine test, but it may be run as part of a chemistry panel.

It should be considered under the following circumstances:

- When kidney stones are present
- When a doctor suspects acute arthritis caused by gout, but has not yet diagnosed the condition
- Leukemia that requires chemotherapy

A full workup may include testing for uric acid in both the blood and by means of a twenty-four-hour urine collection.

BLOOD IMMUNOGLOBULINS

Immunoglobulins are antibodies that help fight disease. They are made by lymphocytes, a type of white blood cell, and require a diet with a good source of protein and a healthy liver for their production.

Immunoglobulin tests are not routine. They are usually performed for the following reasons:

- To test for a specific immunoglobulin, such as rhematoid factor in rheumatoid arthritis
- When low immunoglobulin levels are suspected, as in cases of frequent bacterial infection, or liver or kidney disease
- To measure an immune response such an allergic reaction or to determine whether the immune system is healthy or diseased, such as where AIDS is suspected (see page 213)
- To check for elevated levels of immunoglobulin when such problems as multiple myeloma, a kind of bone tumor, are suspected

BLOOD ANTIBODY TESTS

These tests attempt to detect the presence of particular antibodies in your blood. They are most often used to detect whether or not you have been exposed to a certain virus, since viruses are smaller than bacteria, more difficult to identify, and harder to grow in a culture.

The tests are limited in application for the following reasons:

- Antibodies may not show up until weeks or months after infection (a major problem with AIDS testing; see page 213).
- The tests may take weeks to yield results.
- The tests usually indicate only that you've been exposed to the virus and may be unable to differentiate between exposure in the distant past and recent infection.

This problem is sometimes solvable in the following way: Two separate tests are taken, a number of weeks apart. If the antibody level is much higher during one of those tests, it may indicate that a new infection occurred at that time. However, this method has only been proven accurate for a few viruses and bacteria.

● A large percentage of the population may have been exposed to the virus in question. This is the case with Epstein-Barr virus, for which 50 percent of the population has antibodies. The virus received a great deal of media attention as the possible cause of "chronic fatigue syndrome," but antibody tests were unable to prove a consistent link.

BLOOD TESTS FOR "CONNECTIVE TISSUE DISEASES"

When your body is infected or invaded, your immune system protects you by making antibodies. However, under certain conditions, which may be related to heredity and precipitated by infection, environment, or other factors, the immune system goes awry, and starts making antibodies against your own body.

When this happens, the syndromes collectively referred to as connective tissue disorders (CTD's) may occur. They include rheumatoid arthritis, systemic lupus erythematosus ("lupus" or SLE), and scleroderma. Certain other diseases, such as diabetes, are also believed to be partially due to this phenomenon.

Each of the CTD's is diagnosed by a number of specific blood tests. Rheumatoid arthritis has the rheumatoid factor, while SLE has the LE test and the ANA test (anti-nuclear-antibody, which may also be present in other CTD's).

The tests are anything but routine. They are performed only when your primary-care physician or a rheumatologist, who specializes in these disorders, suspects that you may have a connective tissue disease.

HISTOCOMPATIBILITY TESTING

Histocompatibility tests, also known as HLA for "human leucocyte antigen," are done by studying the chromosomes in the white blood cells. Such tests are performed prior to a transplant operation to determine whether the tissues of prospective donors and recipients are compatible.

"Histocompatibility areas" have been identified on our sixth chromosome; they are examined by electron microscope and other diagnostic techniques. The more similar areas recipient and donor have, the greater the likelihood that the tissue will be accepted.

TUMOR MARKERS

Tumor markers refer to specific biochemicals in the blood that may directly indicate the presence of a tumor. They occur in many different forms, and although some have proved useful in the treatment and early detection of cancer, many others have proved useless.

Oncofetal Antigens

These chemicals occur in fetal tissue, but are almost entirely absent in healthy adults. The discovery of alfa-fetoprotein (AFP) in the blood of patients with liver tumors and cinoembryonic antigen (CEA) in patients with intestinal cancer raised scientists' hopes that these substances might turn out to be ideal screening tests for these cancers. Unfortunately, this has not turned out to be uniformly the case.

CEA has not proven specific or sensitive enough to be used as a screening test—it would miss too many cancers. It has, however, been used with some success to follow a patient's response to treatment. Once a baseline level is measured, increased levels indicate poor response or spread of the tumor, while decreased levels suggest a good response.

AFP is produced not only by liver tumors, but by cancers of the intestine, lung, and testicle as well, so it's also not specific enough for use as a screening test for cancer. (See page 133 for a discussion of AFP as a screening test for fetal abnormalities.) However, it may be used along with human chorionic gonadotrophin (HCG—see below) to monitor patients with testicular tumors.

Human Chorionic Gonadotrophin

Human chorionic gonadotrophin is probably the most accurate tumor marker currently used for screening. This substance is normally made in the developing placenta and disappears in the adult unless certain tumors, including some that affect the lung, the breast, the ovary, the testicles, and the skin (particularly melanoma) begin to grow.

It can be used to detect testicular tumors before they are found on physical exam, and it is already being used fairly accurately to follow the treatment and response of some other cancers.

Prostate-Specific Antigen

PSA is a new tumor marker which shows promise for monitoring the treatment of prostate cancer. Its levels double when the disease has spread and drop when treatment is successful. Initial studies on its ability to screen for undetected cancer are not as promising. Levels are the same for benign enlargement of the prostate as they are for cancer.

There are a number of other tumor markers, none of which has proved to be a perfect screening test. Some, like PSA or AFP, can be used to follow treatment, while many others are still being studied.

A Note on Tumor Markers

Sound confusing? It is, because the field of tumor markers is just developing. The American Cancer Society has made the following statements in an attempt to clarify the current status of the field:

1. Virtually no tumor marker has been shown to be specific or sensitive enough to use for early cancer detection on the general population.
2. At the present time, the main function of tumor markers is to confirm the diagnosis of cancer or to follow the course of treatment.

In light of those statements, you should not ask your doctor to use any of these tests to "screen you for cancer," but you may want to ask if there is a safe, reliable blood test that can monitor your treatment if you develop cancer.

BLOOD TESTS FOR MONONUCLEOSIS

Mononucleosis is really a number of viral diseases that cause the mononuclear white blood cells in your bloodstream to multiply. In the United States, it is most often caused by the Epstein-Barr virus, and the most common two tests for "mono" attempt to detect exposure to that virus.

The *mono-spot* test is reported only as positive or negative.

The *heterophile-antibody* test is the more precise of the two, measuring the concentration of antibodies present.

You may want to have the tests done if you have symptoms of mono such as persistent aches, tiredness, slight sore throat, fevers, and abdominal pain. However, keep in mind that you are only being tested for exposure, not acute infection (see antibody tests, page 204).

HUMAN GROWTH HORMONE (HGH)

Three different abnormalities can affect the normal production of human growth hormone (HGH) and produce medical problems.

- If HGH is too high in childhood, it may cause your child to grow too quickly and too large.
- If HGH is low or absent it may result in dwarfism.
- If HGH increases during adulthood, because of a pituitary tumor, for example, facial bones alone may grow, causing distorted features and a condition called acromegaly.

The blood HGH level should be tested whenever a child exhibits slower or more rapid growth than expected, or when the doctor suspects a pituitary tumor in an adult.

HEART ENZYME TESTS

When heart tissue is injured, its enzymes "leak" into the bloodstream. These enzymes, called creatine phosphokinase (CPK), serum glutamic oxaloacetic transaminase (SGOT), and lactate dehydrogenase (LDH), are usually present in the blood under normal circumstances, but precisely timed tests for measuring increased levels may confirm a diagnosis of heart attack.

The blood samples should be drawn three times in the first day after the development of chest pain and once or twice a day for a week or so thereafter.

If a heart attack has occurred, the CPK level will increase first, followed by the other two. All three enzymes are made elsewhere in the body as well, but special new tests called isoenzyme assays have been developed to determine whether the enzymes tested come from the heart. The blood tests can rarely produce a diagnosis on their own, but when coupled with electrocardiogram and physical examination, they are considered extremely accurate.

BLOOD BILIRUBIN

Bilirubin is a substance that is formed when the hemoglobin in your red blood cells breaks down. It then passes through the bloodstream to the liver (bilirubin on its way to the liver is called "indirect bilirubin"), where it is processed into a more soluble form ("direct bilirubin"), and then excreted into your stool. It is not normally found in urine, and only very small amounts are detectable in blood.

If something happens to increase the breakdown of red blood cells (a "hemolytic anemia"), the level of indirect bilirubin increases in your blood. If the liver cells are damaged or blocked, the direct bilirubin increases. In either case, when the level gets high enough, your skin may turn yellow, a condition commonly called jaundice.

Tests for bilirubin in the blood are not done routinely. They should only be performed to determine the cause of jaundice or abdominal pain, or in the evaluation of hepatitis, unexplained anemia, or pancreatic or gall bladder disease.

ALKALINE PHOSPHATASE

Alkaline phosphatase is an enzyme normally found in your blood. It increases when your liver or bones are damaged. (Levels may also be elevated in healthy growing children.)

The test is not routine. It is used in the diagnosis and monitoring of suspected liver or bone disease, which may result in symptoms such as jaundice or bone and abdominal pain. It is also used to monitor the effects of medications that may be toxic to the liver.

When used in conjunction with tests for bilirubin, amylase, and liver enzymes, it can help to differentiate among problems of the gallbladder, liver, and pancreas.

AMYLASE

Amylase is an enzyme produced by your internal organs, including your salivary glands, liver, pancreas, and a woman's fallopian tubes.

It is not tested routinely, but may be present in elevated levels in diseases that affect any one of the above organs. It is used most often to diagnose pancreatitis, a painful inflammation of the pancreas that can have a variety of causes but is often due to excess alcohol ingestion. An amylase test may also be performed to aid in the evaluation of undiagnosed abdominal pain.

Although higher levels of amylase may indicate problems in any one of several organs, a severe elevation could indicate perforation of the abdominal lining or obstruction of the intestine, both of which require rapid emergency treatment.

LIVER ENZYMES

The two liver enzymes most often tested for are serum glutamic oxaloacetic transaminase (SGOT) and serum glutamic pyruvic transaminase (SGPT). These substances are released into the bloodstream when the liver is affected by injury, infection, or inflammation. Their levels may be elevated as a result of medications that cause harm to the liver and that have been taken as part of the treatment for hepatitis, gallbladder disease, or liver, pancreatic, or gallbladder tumor.

Although SGOT is also found in heart muscles, high levels plus comparison of SGOT levels with SGPT levels may help diagnose the cause of liver problems. When the tests are performed in concert with amylase, alkaline phosphatase, and bilirubin tests, they may help your doctor to narrow down the cause of abdominal pain and jaundice.

SODIUM CHLORIDE TEST FOR CYSTIC FIBROSIS IN THE CHILD (THE SWEAT TEST)

Cystic fibrosis is a congenital disease that causes a chemical alteration in many of the body's glands. This alteration affects the child's ability to breathe, perspire, and eat. It may result in frequent lung infections, poor growth, poor nutrition, and early death. Early diagnosis, which this test may provide, can reduce the complications and prolong life.

Electrodes are attached to the child's arm and a painless electrical current is passed through the skin as medication is applied to the area to increase the child's perspiration. The electrodes are then removed and a special collecting paper is placed over the spot. Less than an hour later, the paper is removed and evaluated for sodium and chloride. Abnormally high levels of these elements provide the diagnosis and allow the implementation of preventive steps to treat the child.

Body fluid tests are rarely dangerous and they may lead your doctor to early diagnosis and cure of a problem that might otherwise prove life-threatening. Most of them are nowhere near as elaborate as the sweat test described above. However, because they are so simple to perform and because we are so prevention-minded, they are among the most overused tests in our medical tool chest. Beware of unscrupulous laboratories that offer "preventive screening tests" without mentioning whether or not your insurance will pay for them, and of well-meaning doctors who lack the experience to be selective.

Make sure you get the tests that are listed as routine for your age group in Chapter Six. If a doctor or clinic suggests some other test on your body fluid, read its description here and discuss with your doctor whether or not you really need it before having it performed. Don't hesitate to get a second or even a third opinion. You'll save yourself a lot of needless anxiety and cost while promoting your continued health.

FIFTEEN

Tests for Sexually Transmitted Diseases (STD's)

A few years ago, a patient came to my office with a sad, frustrating story. She was only 29 years old, but she had already been through six of the most painful, frustrating years you could imagine—emotionally as well as physically.

Her problems began when she was 23. Her boyfriend caught gonorrhea, but since he didn't inform her, they continued to have sexual relations. She never developed symptoms, so when the boyfriend had a relapse six months later and finally admitted his problem to her, she didn't visit her doctor. The first time she sought help was the following year, when she noticed tender blisters on her genital area and developed severe pelvic pain.

The sores turned out to be herpes and the pain was due to a "tubal pregnancy" (see page 126). As it turns out, she had caught gonorrhea from her boyfriend and, although it caused her no symptoms, it infected and scarred her fallopian tubes. The tubal pregnancy occurred because the healthy embryo couldn't get past the scars to reach her uterus. She needed life-saving surgery to remove the pregnancy, but she feared she'd never conceive again.

After breaking up with her boyfriend, she met a man, fell in love, and got married. To her surprise and delight, she became pregnant within a year. However, she developed a recurrence of the herpes infection just before delivery and required an emergency caesarean section to protect the baby from catching the infection.

That baby did fine, but she and her new husband had since then been unable to conceive, and she came to me because her fears about infertility had resurfaced.

This story is completely true, and all too common. The saddest part is that both infections and the subsequent problems could have been prevented by a little knowledge and communication.

The subject may be embarrassing, the need to check for exposure even more so, but your understanding of the tests for sexually transmitted diseases (STD's) is crucial for your own health and for the health of your loved ones.

- AIDS now affects more than 40,000 people in the United States. It's a tragic disease, but it's not the only STD to have reached epidemic proportions.
- Gonorrhea is more common today than it was a few decades ago, and more cases are resistant to penicillin.
- Incidence of syphilis has increased by 30 percent in the past few years.
- Venereal warts have been shown to increase the risk of cervical cancer in women.
- Chlamydia, now the most common STD, is capable of causing infertility.

The situation sounds ominous, but the spread of these diseases can be controlled.

Keep the following crucial rules about the control and prevention of STD's in mind:

1. If you have had sexual contact with someone who later informs you that they have an STD, make sure you are tested, even if you don't have any symptoms.
2. If you develop symptoms yourself, don't wait. Read the section on that STD test and consider having it done.
3. Whenever you are tested for one STD, consider testing for the others as well. The diseases often coexist, and studies have shown that they're related biologically. Infection with one may make you socially and physically more susceptible to the others.
4. If you develop symptoms or test positive for an STD, make sure all of your recent (within the past year) sexual contacts know.

   In the case of AIDS, you may have to notify all contacts from more than the past ten years.

STD tests are not necessary for everyone, but you can protect yourself and your loved ones by learning when they should be done and how to interpret the results. Read the description of each test below.

THE TESTS FOR AIDS

AIDS is not an infection; it is the result of an infection.

Acquired immunodeficiency syndrome (AIDS) occurs when a virus, now called the human immunodeficiency virus (HIV), attacks the immunological system and renders its victim helpless against certain infections and cancers.

The virus is spread most often by sexual contact, but may be spread by contaminated blood or needles. It is not spread by saliva, sweat, tears, urine, or bowel movements, and you cannot get it by kissing or holding hands.

The two major tests that check for exposure to the HIV are called the ELISA or EIA (for enzyme immunoassay) and the Western blot. Other tests include the RIP (for Radioimmunoprecipitation test) and IFA (for Immunofluorescent Antibody test). These tests check for antibodies to the virus; if the blood harbors antibodies, it is proof of exposure. Usually, it takes anywhere from six to twelve weeks to develop antibodies, but they have been reported as early as three weeks and as late as eighteen months after exposure.

The decision of whether or not to have a test for AIDS is understandably fraught with confusion and fear, but it is a crucial decision that *must* be made.

What Is the Purpose of the Tests?

An AIDS test checks for the presence of antibodies. If they are present, it means that the person has, at some time in the past, been infected by the virus.

Such results are significant, since they tell the patient that he or she is capable of infecting someone else, and they allow the doctor to consider the need for early treatment or other measures to help stave off the development of AIDS. Since it may take six weeks or longer for the antibodies to appear, it is possible to be infected and test negative.

How Are the Tests Performed?

In all cases, a small sample of blood is taken from an arm vein. During an ELISA test, this blood is added to small amounts of dead AIDS virus in a test kit. If the blood sample contains antibodies to the virus, they will attach themselves to the dead virus particles, and the test samples will turn a distinctive color. A positive test is almost always repeated. If the second is also positive, a different test, called the Western blot, is used to confirm the results. The Western blot is more precise than the ELISA because it attempts to detect small parts of the virus rather than the whole virus. A few labs offer other tests, and some are now working on methods to detect the virus itself, but these two are currently used most often because of their reliability, rapid results (within a few days), and low cost. The ELISA may cost only one dollar, the Western blot thirty to seventy dollars.

Where and by Whom Should the Tests Be Performed and Interpreted?

AIDS tests are performed at a number of hospitals and clinics throughout the country, or your doctor may be able to draw the blood himself and send it to a special lab. For the testing center nearest you, call your local AIDS hotline, or call 1-800-342-AIDS.

Your doctor can read the lab results to you, but because of the dangers of misinterpreting the results or misunderstanding their implications, positive findings should always be evaluated by an expert in the diagnosis and treatment of AIDS. This usually means an internist with special training in infectious disease and/or immunology and with special experience in dealing with AIDS.

How Accurate Are These Tests?

The combination of the ELISA and Western blot tests has been described as "among the best tests ever developed for any viral infection."

Still, their interpretation in the case of positive or indeterminate findings requires the cooperation of a licensed experienced lab and a doctor who is an expert in the diagnosis and treatment of AIDS.

The ELISA has been estimated to be about 98 percent accurate in high-risk groups and slightly less accurate in those at low risk. By itself, the Western blot is more specific. It will help weed out a few false positives, but it is more complex and takes more experience to interpret. On occasion, it may be reported as "indeterminate" and need to be repeated within a few weeks. When the two tests are combined, the overall accuracy approaches 99 percent.

Still, experts report as many as 11 false positives, and 2 false negatives per 100,000 people tested. There's also the small but real possibility that the infection is present but antibodies have not yet appeared. For all of these reasons, it is imperative that the results be discussed with an expert.

What Are the Dangers of Doing the Tests?

All blood tests carry a small risk of infection or bleeding around the puncture site. The AIDS tests carry the additional profound danger of misinterpretation.

Someone who receives a false-positive result will think he has been exposed to the HIV virus when in fact he hasn't. This mistake can cause a great deal of trauma, uncertainty, and unnecessary and costly medical care.

Someone who receives a false-negative result is likely to be lulled into a false sense of security. He may not only fail to receive appropriate treatment, but also infect others with the virus.

These dangers can all be minimized by making sure that you get the test only if it's necessary, and that it's interpreted by an expert.

Are the Tests Really Necessary?

The question of who should be tested for AIDS has become a legal and moral issue as well as a medical one. For our purposes, we'll focus only on the medical issues. Keeping in mind that testing people at high risk increases the accuracy of the test, experts list the following people in that category:

- Homosexual men and bisexual men who are not intravenous drug users
- Intravenous drug users, regardless of sexual practices. Homosexual or bisexual men who are intravenous drug users are at even higher risk
- Heterosexual contacts of the above groups
- Patients who received blood transfusions between 1978 and mid-1985
- Hemophilia patients

While sexual contact with anyone in the above high-risk groups may place you at risk and lead to a definite need for an AIDS test, the decision to have one performed under other circumstances is often more difficult. It can get confusing, and frightening. To alleviate these problems, a number of health services have suggested testing guidelines.

The following is a list of people who, experts generally agree, should be routinely counseled and tested for HIV infection:

- Men who have had sex with other men, especially anal intercourse
- All hemophiliacs
- All persons seeking treatment for other STD's
- All persons seeking treatment for intravenous drug use
- All pregnant women and women of childbearing age who have any of the above identifiable risks of infection

- All prostitutes who seek medical care
- All people being evaluated for signs or symptoms of AIDS, including unexplained, persistent infections or cancers, persistent or serious STD's, chronic, unexplained swelling of lymph nodes, diarrhea, fever, or weight loss

In addition, the following people should be counseled and consider having AIDS testing:

- People who received blood transfusions between early 1978 and mid-1985. Pretransfusion testing of blood since that time has significantly improved.
- People who believe they are at risk for exposure

These guidelines vary from state to state and doctor to doctor. If you're unsure of your own risk level, discuss it with an expert.

WHAT SHOULD YOU DO IF YOU GET A NEGATIVE RESULT?

Remember that it is possible to test negative in spite of infection, if your exposure has been recent. The danger zone is six to twelve weeks, but on a rare occasion, it has taken eighteen months for the antibodies to appear. The advice is simple:

If you're unsure, repeat the test at an appropriate time after your last questionable exposure.

If this second test is negative and/or you and your partner have been monogamous for eighteen months and you have no risk factors, you're absolutely safe.

WHAT SHOULD YOU DO IF YOU GET A POSITIVE RESULT?

1. Have the test repeated.
2. Discuss the situation with an expert.
3. If it is determined that you are positive, take the following steps:
   - Inform all of your sexual contacts over the course of at least the past ten years. They should be tested, as should your children, if you have any.
   - Do not donate blood to a blood bank or semen to a semen bank, as either may carry the infection.
   - Abstain from sex or practice "safe sex" from that point on, since you are now capable of spreading the virus.
   - If you are a woman of childbearing age, before you get pregnant, consider the fact that 20 to 50 percent of women who have tested positive have passed the infection on to their unborn child.

● Understand that a positive test means that you have been infected with the virus. It does not mean that you have AIDS.

Although experts fear that a large majority, if not all, of those people who have been infected will develop AIDS, new and better treatments are being developed every day.

Since research has proved that early treatment prolongs and improves the quality of life, make sure you get regular checkups with an expert in the diagnosis and treatment of AIDS.

OTHER STD'S

Gonorrhea, syphilis, herpes, venereal warts, and chlamydia urethritis are transmitted mainly by sexual contact. They also share two other characteristics that make their diagnosis elusive and their spread pandemic:

● They may not cause initial symptoms (this is especially true for women).
● When they do, the symptoms may disappear without treatment while the infection continues.

In either case, the person without symptoms may still be capable of infecting other people. Also, the diseases may remain active, causing serious, irreversible damage to the internal organs.

For those reasons, it's important that you understand when and why each test is necessary, and it is crucial that you follow the guidelines for the detection and prevention of STD's:

1. If you have had sexual contact with a person known or suspected to have an STD, you should be tested, whether or not you have symptoms.
2. The suspicion or diagnosis of any STD should lead to a test for the other STD's as well, since they often coexist and infection with one may predispose you to catching the others.
3. If you test positive, you should notify all people with whom you have had sexual contact. Unlike AIDS, the other STD's require that you notify only recent contacts, such as those from the preceding year.

GONORRHEA

Gonorrhea is caused by a bacterium called *Neisseria gonorrheae*. It often causes urinary discharge or discomfort, but symptoms may be mild or absent, especially in the woman.

If it is caught in this first stage it's easily treatable, but if left untreated it can cause serious problems, including pelvic inflammatory disease (PID, an illness that causes acute pelvic pain and fever), life-threatening tubal pregnancies, scarred fallopian tubes, which could cause infertility, and what is commonly called "disseminated gonorrhea." In this last form, gonorrhea infects the blood and joints, and can infect other organs, causing fever and joint pain. This complication is not as rare as you might think. The most common cause of a hot, swollen, red knee in an otherwise healthy young person who has no history of knee injury is disseminated gonorrhea.

What Is the Purpose of the Test?

Gonorrhea tests are done simply to determine whether an infection is being caused by the bacterium *Neisseria gonorrheae,* so that it may be properly treated.

How Is the Test Performed?

When discharge is present, it can be sampled and cultured to test for the bacteria.

In the man, this involves the sterile cleaning of the meatus (the external opening of the penis) and the insertion of a cotton swab to obtain a sample for microscopic examination and culture.

In the woman, the same procedure may be undertaken on her meatus, but more than 95 percent of women have no discharge. As a result, a pelvic exam is usually necessary. In that case, the samples are taken from the cervix and vagina.

If disseminated gonorrhea occurs, the blood will also have to be tested repeatedly for signs of bacterial infection, and antibiotics will have to be given intravenously.

Where and by Whom Should the Test Be Performed and Interpreted?

Your primary-care physician or gynecologist or an emergency physician can perform the test, which either he or the laboratory pathologist can then interpret. In cases of disseminated gonorrhea, an infectious disease expert may have to be called in.

How Accurate Is the Test?

If discharge is present, the test is very accurate, but if it is not, the test may be useless. Also, while a positive finding is clear evidence that the disease exists, a negative finding may mean that the doctor has to base the diagnosis and treatment on his best educated guess.

In any case, a negative test should lead your doctor to test for other causes of discharge, including chlamydia (see page 223).

What Are the Dangers of the Test?

There are no dangers with the cotton swab test.

The blood tests carry the same slight risk as any test that involves the use of a needle: infection or bleeding at the puncture site.

Is It Really Necessary?

The tests are not meant for routine screening. But they are absolutely necessary whenever you develop discharge or have had sexual contact with someone who is suspected of having gonorrhea.

SYPHILIS

Syphilis is also caused by a bacterium—one called *Treponema pallidum.*

The development of penicillin, which is capable of eradicating the disease in its early stages, helped control the disease in the past. However, there has been a 30 percent increase in its spread recently, so it is now more crucial than ever that you understand both the disease process and the tests that check for its presence.

When the bacterium enters the body, it usually causes a "chancre" sore—a painless, red, raised bump near the site of entry—within three weeks.

This sore will disappear, whether or not the disease is treated.

Up to six months later, a red, raised rash appears, most often on the hands and feet, but occasionally over the back and trunk as well.

This, too, will disappear without treatment.

The final stage, which can affect the heart, brain, and spinal cord, may not occur until one or two decades later. At this point, it may cause death or irreversible damage—and both diagnosis and treatment may prove more difficult.

Your understanding of this sequence of symptoms and of the tests used to detect syphilis will help to prevent those complications from occurring.

What Is the Purpose of the Tests?

These tests seek to determine whether or not you have been exposed to syphilis.

How Are the Tests Performed?

When chancre sores are present, bacteria can be obtained for identification. The sores are scraped with a needle or blade to obtain a cell sample, which is then examined for the presence of the characteristic spiral-shaped bacteria. A special "dark-field" microscope must be used, because the syphilis-causing bacterium is difficult to see.

VDRL (Venereal Disease Research Laboratory) is a blood test that checks for the presence of substances which prove that the patient has been exposed to the infection.

FTA-ABS (Fluorescent Treponemal Antibody Absorption) is also a blood test that seeks to detect evidence of exposure, but it is used only to confirm the infection when the VDRL or RPR is positive.

Where and by Whom Should the Tests Be Performed and Interpreted?

Dark-field microscopy should be performed and interpreted by a physician who has experience in such examinations. In many circumstances, this will require an infectious disease expert or dermatologist to assist with the scraping and either of them or a pathologist to do the interpretation.

The blood tests can be drawn by a technician, a nurse, or a doctor. Because they test different stages of infection and must be used at different intervals after exposure, your doctor may (or may not, if he has the experience himself) require a specialist's help for interpretation.

How Accurate Are the Tests?

The microscopic examination is very accurate when chancres are present.

The VDRL and RPR tests may prove "false negative," missing one out of four infections, early in the disease, but are more accurate later on.

The FTA-ABS test is extremely accurate, but it doesn't work until about a month after the initial infection. The sequence of tests may therefore be crucial to correct diagnosis (see below).

What Are the Dangers of Doing the Tests?

The only danger is the slight possibility of local infection or bleeding at the scraping or puncture sites.

Are the Tests Really Necessary?

Dark-field microscopy is necessary whenever there is a history of exposure and a chancre appears.

VDRL and RPR are routine screening tests that should be done once after the age of 18 and repeated whenever exposure is suspected. In those circumstances, if they are negative, and you are concerned that they were done too early to detect evidence of infection, they should be repeated at an appropriate later date.

FTA-ABS tests are done whenever VDRL or RPR are positive.

Although each test has its limitations, the proper sequence and interpretation can ensure accurate diagnosis and appropriate treatment.

HERPES

Herpes infections are caused by two viruses, herpes simplex virus 1 or herpes simplex virus 2 (HSV1 or HSV2). Although HSV1 more often causes facial sores and HSV2 more often affects the genitals, either virus is capable of infecting both areas.

Herpes is an example of a latent infection. After the initial infection, it is beaten back but is not eradicated. It remains buried within the body (usually in a nerve root) and causes symptoms from time to time whenever the immune system lets its guard down, because of other infections, stress, poor nutrition, or other unknown factors.

The first sores usually appear within three weeks of exposure, and there usually are repeat episodes at various times throughout life. There may be a long latent period between the first and second sets of symptoms—as long as decades; and some people have recurrent episodes for five years, then never experience another attack. The course is individual and variable and tests for the problem are not always accurate. For those reasons, diagnosis may have to be based on history and symptoms, rather than laboratory findings.

However it's made, diagnosis is important. Mothers are capable of passing the virus on to their children if the infection is active during delivery. Herpes has been associated with an increased risk of cervical cancer in women. Also, although latent carriers go through long, noninfectious periods, there are times when it is possible for them to spread the infection despite the apparent absence of the characteristic sores.

What Is the Purpose of the Tests?

The tests are done to confirm a suspected diagnosis. As with all STD tests, it may also be performed when other STD tests are positive, to check for coexisting exposure.

How Are the Tests Performed?

When the sores are present, they may be scraped or drained, then sent to a special laboratory for microscopic examination and culture.

The blood test for antibodies is drawn as are all other blood samples. It is then sent to a laboratory, which reports the findings to your doctor within a period of about two weeks.

Where and by Whom Should the Tests Be Performed and Interpreted?

Your primary doctor or a dermatologist can perform the tests and do the initial scraping and microscopic examination, but he will then send it to a special laboratory or pathologist for definitive interpretation.

How Accurate Are the Tests?

Microscopic examination is highly inaccurate. It is very possible to have herpes and have this test turn out negative.

The laboratory culture tests (see page 156 for an explanation of cultures) are far more accurate, especially when performed and interpreted by an expert. Unfortunately, improper collection is common and seriously increases the chance of a false negative.

Even under ideal circumstances, however, it is possible to have herpes and be unable to detect it by laboratory test. These false negatives are not unusual, but false positives (getting a positive result when you don't have the infection) are rare.

What Are the Dangers of the Tests?

The only dangers are those of local infection or bleeding.

Are They Really Necessary?

The diagnosis of herpes infection is a clinical one, based on your symptoms and the doctor's examination. Keep in mind that the tests may be inaccurate and that treatment is noncurative. It will subdue the infection and symptoms, but to date no way has been found to completely wipe out the virus.

For these reasons, the tests are not always necessary. They may be appropriate under the following circumstances:

- Whenever diagnosis is uncertain
- Whenever serious infections, such as those that spread to more than one area, are present

CHLAMYDIA

Chlamydia trachomatis is an organism that is larger than a virus but smaller than a bacterium.

Chlamydia is the most common STD in the United States. Like gonorrhea, it may not cause symptoms in the woman, and if left untreated, it can lead to serious complications. It may be passed from mother to unborn child, cause serious pelvic infections, infertility, life-threatening tubal pregnancies, visual problems, and pneumonia.

Diagnosis is simple, but it is only accurate when the infection is suspected, and the specific tests are ordered. Chlamydia is easily missed, and if the wrong antibiotic is chosen, serious complications may ensue. (For a fictionalized example of such a possibility, see page 19).

What Is the Purpose of the Test?

Chlamydia is easily treated, usually with the antibiotic tetracycline. If it's missed, however, it is easily spread, and the epidemic continues. This specific test can halt that spread and prevent the complications.

How Is the Test Performed?

In the past, the entire organism itself had to be identified, but now there is a simpler, less expensive, and more accurate test that checks for part of the organism. Fluid is taken from the urethra through the external opening above the vagina or at end of the penis or from the cervix during a pelvic exam, then sent to a special lab for examination and culture. The lab slip must specifically request that the specimen be tested for chlamydia.

How Accurate Is the Test?

When the specific test is requested of the laboratory, the diagnosis is correctly made in nearly 90 percent of cases; fewer than 15 percent are missed, and only 5 percent test false positive.

When the test is not requested and the fluid is examined only for other organisms, a missed diagnosis is far more likely.

What Are the Dangers of the Test?

Aside from mild discomfort during the test, there are no dangers.

Is the Test Really Necessary?

One study showed that nearly one out of ten women who did not have symptoms but were routinely tested during a pelvic exam turned out to have evidence of chlamydial infection. As a result, some experts have suggested routine examinations of women for chlamydia, but others have argued that it's not cost-effective.

The current consensus is that the following people, who are most at risk for the infection, should have the test performed:

- Anyone who has a genital discharge
- Anyone who complains of urinary discomfort and is suspected of having an STD
- Anyone diagnosed as having one of the other STD's
- Anyone who has had sexual contact with someone who has been diagnosed as having an STD

In addition, some experts have suggested that women who have at least two of the following five risk factors should consider having the test.

- Age younger than 25
- Intercourse with a new partner within the past two months
- Genital discharge
- Cervical bleeding
- Regular intercourse with different partners without the use of a condom, diaphragm, or cervical cap

Despite the fact that chlamydia is our most common STD, tests are performed for its detection far less commonly than for many of the other STD's.

In the past, this has been true because of the cost of various tests and because of the lack of a specific test for diagnosis.

Since one now exists, and others are being developed, the tests may soon be recommended on a more routine basis.

VENEREAL WARTS

Venereal warts or *Condylomata accuminata* is a sexually transmitted disease that is believed to be caused by the human papilloma virus; they have been associated with an increased risk of cervical cancer in women. They may be apparent on physical exam, but they are sometimes invisible to the human eye.

You should look for them on your own physical, and your doctor should look for them every time he performs an examination in him office. They should be suspected of existing (whether or not they're visible) in the following cases:

- Exposure to someone with a known history of venereal warts
- Exposure to someone who has been diagnosed as having an STD
- In women who have undiagnosed cervical bleeding, an abnormal Pap smear, or abnormal cervical appearance on a pelvic exam
- In men whose sex partner has venereal warts or develops an abnormal Pap smear or cervical cancer

For these high-risk people, colposcopy (see page 121) may be considered if the warts are not visible on a physical exam. As with any STD, a positive diagnosis should lead to tests for other STD's and the notification of all sexual contacts.

Sexually transmitted diseases have a social and emotional stigma attached to them. No one likes to talk about them, and many people would rather not even consider the possibility that they've been exposed.

That's understandable, but don't let such fears make you ignore symptoms or a history of exposure. STD's won't go away without treatment, even if their symptoms do.

They are serious, highly infectious diseases that can lead to infertility and death if they remain undetected. In most cases, the tests for their presence are simple and the treatment highly effective. This is one place where your knowledge and participation can mean the difference between health and severe illness—for yourself and for your loved ones.

Sixteen

Miscellaneous Tests

Of the following five tests, which don't fall into any of the categories described in Chapters Seven through Fifteen, only glaucoma testing is routine. It needs to be performed on a regular basis, even if you don't have symptoms. See Chapter Six to determine when you should have the test performed.

The other four tests may be required if your doctor suspects that you have one of the problems they test for. In those cases, they will provide valuable diagnostic information and may help your doctor to plan your treatment.

ELECTROENCEPHALOGRAM (EEG)

What Is the Purpose of the Test?

Disturbances in brain waves can help to pick up subtle changes that may not be apparent on other examinations or tests. EEG's are used to diagnose seizures, to investigate sleep disorders and periods of unconsciousness, and for legal purposes—to confirm brain death in comatose patients.

How Is the Test Performed?

The EEG is performed by placing electrodes on your scalp, then recording the tiny electrical impulses that are your brain waves.

Where and by Whom Should the Test Be Performed and Interpreted?

The EEG is usually administered in a clinic, office, or hospital. A specially trained EEG technician should perform the test, and a specialized neurologist should evaluate the results.

How Accurate Is the Test?

EEG's are very accurate for the detection of seizure focuses (the areas in the brain where the seizure originates) and for the evaluation of coma and unconsciousness. They may detect early changes in other brain disorders, such as tumor or infection, but they are rarely as precise or as specific as CAT scans and MRI's for those purposes.

What Are the Dangers of Doing the Test?

There is almost no risk associated with EEG's.

Is It Really Necessary?

This is not a routine test, but it may be ordered for the following reasons:

- To diagnose seizures and find out what part of the brain they're coming from
- To evaluate unconsciousness or coma
- To evaluate sleep disorders
- In addition to other tests, to make a diagnosis of certain brain or nervous system disorders

SLEEP APNEA TESTING

If your partner snores at night, but is sleepy during the day, he or she may have "sleep apnea." This condition is caused either by a problem in the central nervous system or by a subtle and partial blockage in the back of the throat. It results in periods of time when less than adequate oxygen reaches the brain. As a result, the person is tired the next day, despite an apparently restful night.

There are treatments for the disorder, which most often affects obese people and those with high blood pressure, but diagnosis can only be achieved if the condition is suspected and tested for.

What Is the Purpose of the Test?

The test is performed to check for sleep apnea or to evaluate daytime sleepiness. It may also be used to evaluate the possibility of narcolepsy, a nervous system disorder that causes sudden, unexplained periods of loss of consciousness during the day.

How Is the Test Performed?

Sleep apnea testing can only be performed during sleep. You are checked into a clinic or a hospital, connected to an EEG machine and videotaped while you sleep. The entire time, a machine called an oximeter, which is attached to your ear lobe or tiny finger, will monitor the level of oxygen in your blood. The EEG, videotape, and oxygen measurements will then be evaluated by an expert.

Where and by Whom Should the Test Be Performed and Interpreted?

Sleep apnea tests are usually done in a hospital or clinic and must be interpreted by an expert in the evaluation of sleep apnea.

How Accurate Is the Test?

This test is virtually foolproof for the detection of sleep apnea.

What Are the Dangers of Doing the Test?

There are no dangers, save the slight risk of infection or local bleeding if blood tests are used to measure oxygen.

Is It Really Necessary?

This test is not routine; it is complex and expensive and should only be done on appropriate people. Because it is safe, accurate, and noninvasive, however, it may be undertaken on those who are suspected of having sleep apnea or some other sleeping disorder.

It is especially indicated for people who have all of the risk factors for sleep apnea: snoring, high blood pressure, obesity, and complaints of daytime sleepiness.

ALLERGY TESTING

Allergies occur when the immune system overreacts to otherwise harmless foreign substances such as pollens or certain foods.

What Is the Purpose of the Tests?

An allergy test is performed to identify the substance (or allergen) that is causing the rash, hay fever, or asthma, so that you can avoid it or receive allergy shots to reduce its effect.

Skin tests are usually used to identify airborne allergens that may be triggering sneezing, a runny nose, nasal congestion, hay fever, or asthma.

Patch tests are more usually used to diagnose unexplained rashes, which may be the result of chemical allergies caused by rubber, nickel, cosmetics, or preservatives. RAST (Radioallergosorbent test) tests seek to diagnose both types of allergies, but they are less specific.

How Are the Tests Performed?

Skin tests are done by scratching or puncturing the skin with a needle that has a small amount of a suspected allergy-producing substance on it.

Patch tests are performed by placing a solution of the material on the skin and leaving it there for up to forty-eight hours.

In both cases, an inflammation at the site of the test indicates that you are allergic to that substance.

RAST tests measure the level in the blood of antibodies to specific allergenic substances.

Where and by Whom Should the Tests Be Performed and Interpreted?

The tests are usually performed and interpreted in the office of a doctor who has been trained in allergy and immunology. A technician or nurse can administer and do a preliminary reading of the test, but the doctor should do the final interpretation.

How Accurate Are the Tests?

Skin and patch tests are more reliable than RAST. But it is possible to have an allergy and not show it on any of these tests. In those cases, if the suspicion of allergy to a specific substance is high, allergy shots may still work to prevent allergic reactions.

What Are the Dangers of Doing the Tests?

Localized itching and swelling are common—they are what the tests seek to detect. More serious reactions such as wheezing or generalized rash occur about 15 percent of the time, but they are easily treated. Extreme, life-threatening allergic reactions ("anaphylactic reactions") are the worst danger, but they are rare, occurring about .05 percent of the time. They, too, can be effectively treated with medications such as epinephrine. Make sure your doctor has experience in treating this possibility.

In both skin and patch tests, there is also the minor risk of local infection at the puncture site. The rare additional danger of a persistent change in skin shade (lighter or darker) exists with the patch test.

Are the Tests Really Necessary?

Allergy testing and allergy shots can help make you more comfortable and in certain extreme circumstances (such as that of a serious drug allergy) save your life. However, since the whole point of an allergy test is to identify the source of the allergy, allergy testing should be considered only in the following circumstances:

- When the cause of a persistent, troublesome allergy has not been diagnosed
- When asthma is persistent and troublesome and an allergy is suspected
- When the cause of a life-threatening allergic reaction has not been identified

In this last circumstance, the testing should be done under very controlled circumstances, possibly in a hospital setting, by an expert who has experience in the emergency treatment of allergic reactions.

PULMONARY FUNCTION TESTS (PFT'S)

What Is the Purpose of These Tests?

Pulmonary function tests are used to diagnose the cause and extent of breathing problems. They help to distinguish among the different forms of lung disease, such as asthma, bronchitis, pulmonary fibrosis, and emphysema.

They may also be used to monitor someone with lung disease over the course of time, or to evaluate the effects of different medications.

How Are the Tests Performed?

Pulmonary function tests are performed by having you breathe into a mouthpiece, then calculating the amounts of air you take in and blow out as well as the times it takes you to perform certain maneuvers.

A variety of tests can be performed. Some of them require deep, slow breathing; others require a sudden, forced puff of air, much as you would use to blow a candle out; and still others are performed after you inhale medication.

Where and by Whom Should the Tests Be Performed and Interpreted?

Some simple pulmonary function tests can be performed at the doctor's office or at your bedside, but complete lung function testing is usually done in a pulmonary function lab or respiratory therapy department.

In those circumstances, they should be done by a specially trained therapist or technician and interpreted by a doctor who specializes in the diagnosis and treatment of lung problems.

How Accurate Are the Tests?

PFT's are the most accurate, precise way to distinguish among many different causes of lung disease.

What Are the Dangers of Doing the Tests?

These tests are safe for most individuals. If you have a severe heart or lung problem, however, they may increase the stress on your heart. If that is the case, discuss the risk involved with your doctor before having the tests performed. In most situations, simple precautions can be taken that will make the test possible while safeguarding your health.

Are the Tests Really Necessary?

PFT's are not routine tests. But they are extremely helpful in the diagnosis of lung problems and are appropriate in the following circumstances:

● To distinguish among various causes of breathing problems when other tests such as a physical exam, blood tests, and a chest x-ray have not produced a diagnosis. They are often used after these other tests as well, to help define the precise diagnosis and plan treatment.

- To follow the course of a certain disease, such as emphysema, in order to choose the most helpful treatment.
- During an acute asthmatic attack, PFT's are used in a limited fashion to determine how severe the attack is and what medications are needed.
- Before chest operations for certain diseases such as lung cancer, to determine whether or not part of or the entire lung can be safely removed.

GLAUCOMA TESTS

One out of every six cases of adult-onset blindness in this country is due to glaucoma, a disease in which pressure inside the eye increases and endangers the nerve that carries images from the retina to the brain.

Early detection and treatment are essential.

What Is the Purpose of the Tests?

Glaucoma tests are performed to detect glaucoma so that it can be treated before it causes damage to your vision.

How Are the Tests Performed?

Simple tonometry is performed by putting some numbing drops into your eye, then placing a small metal instrument called a tonometer onto its surface to determine whether or not your inner eye pressure is too high.

If it is, the *applanation method* may be suggested in order to measure the precise amount of increased pressure.

The doctor will press a special instrument against your cornea while examining it through a magnifying lens. The amount of tension it takes to depress the cornea will give him an accurate measurement of the pressure inside your eye.

The least common, and least accurate, way to check for glaucoma is called the *noncontact method*. In this test, a bright light is shined into your eye, and several brief puffs of air blown into the eye while a machine calculates the pressure within the eye from the changes in the way the cornea reflects the light.

Where and by Whom Should the Tests Be Performed and Interpreted?

An optometrist, ophthalmologist, or family physician can perform simple tonometry in his office.

The applanation method, which requires more expert care, should be performed by an ophthalmologist.

Any questions or an unclear diagnosis should be evaluated by an ophthalmologist, who should be the one to prescribe treatment and follow the patient over the course of time.

How Accurate Are the Tests?

These tests are the definitive ways to diagnose glaucoma. Of the three, the applanation method is the most precise and accurate.

What Are the Dangers of Doing the Tests?

There is minimal risk of eye infection or corneal scratches. These are easily treatable, but could lead to serious problems if ignored. If you feel pain or discomfort after having the test, made sure to have your eyes reexamined.

Are They Really Necessary?

Tests for glaucoma are necessary whenever you have unexplained pain in your eye or whenever your vision becomes impaired.

They are recommended on a routine basis (every three to five years) after the age of 40 and should be performed sooner and more frequently if you have a personal or family history of glaucoma or diabetes.

Black people, who are at increased risk of developing glaucoma, may have to begin testing during their early twenties.

The nonroutine tests, EEG's, sleep apnea testing, allergy testing, and pulmonary function, should be performed only if you develop symptoms or if your doctor suspects that you have a disorder which one of these tests seeks to detect.

If any one of those situations occurs, make sure to read the description of the test and ask all Six Crucial Questions before agreeing to have it performed.

SEVENTEEN
Home Medical Tests

The cost of medical care outside the home has risen more than 300 percent in the past decade—and it promises to rise even higher as medical technology advances and our life expectancy increases. We are living longer than ever before, are more concerned with preventive medicine, and nearly three-quarters of our older generation has some medical condition that requires regular monitoring. It's no wonder that America has taken so quickly to home medical testing.

For a few dollars, you can check yourself for pregnancy, strep throat, diabetes, urinary tract infections, intestinal cancer, gonorrhea and a whole host of other medical conditions without ever leaving the privacy of your home. There are now over one hundred home medical testing kits on the market, and Americans will spend more than $700 million on them in 1989. These safe, relatively inexpensive kits seem to fulfill many of the needs of a modern, health-conscious world:

- Home detection of high blood pressure can lead to early treatment and cut your chance of stroke and heart disease in half.
- Diabetics can monitor their blood and urine sugar levels, help their doctors to keep the disease under control, and prevent complications.
- The American Cancer Society estimates that early detection of cancer of the large intestine by means of home medical tests could double, or even triple, the cure rate. Since blood in the stool is often the first sign of intestinal cancer, the home kit that tests for it could make the difference between life and death.

The kits have their limitations as well, however, and the dangers are not always as apparent. Unless you are aware of them, overreliance on home testing or misinterpretation of the results could prove far worse than never using these tests at all, as the following two examples illustrate.

- A woman who has a tubal pregnancy but gets a negative result on a home test, either because she misread it or because it was too early in the pregnancy to register, might put off going to the doctor, and endanger her life.
- A man whose urinary discharge tests negative for gonorrhea might have some other sexually transmitted disease that the kit does not test for. Because he thinks he's gotten a clean bill of health, he might spread the infection instead of controlling it.

Many of the other kits can lead to similar problems. If you use the tests properly, however, they'll save you money and time, while providing you with the tools to help your doctor prevent, diagnose, and treat disease.

Skim through each of the following sections now. Then, if you buy a home testing kit, review the section on that particular kit carefully and pay close attention to the instructions that come with the kit.

Make sure to follow the general, protective guidelines for home testing that are listed at the end of this chapter.

HOME PREGNANCY TESTS

Home pregnancy tests were first introduced in the 1970's. Today there are many varieties of testing kits available, but they all work on the same principle.

The kits are designed to test for the presence of a hormone called human chorionic gonadotrophin (HCG) in the urine. This hormone is only present in minute amounts during normal life, but it increases during pregnancy because it is produced by the developing placenta. Claims are made by some of the new brands that they can detect this hormone as early as a single day after a missed period, but you may need to allow for a three-day time lag to be sure of the results.

Test your first urine of the day with the pretreated slide or chemically treated piece of paper in the test kit. If the slide or paper changes color, or the urine forms a clump or ring (this varies from brand to brand), your test result is positive.

Time   20 minutes to 2 hours.

Cost $10 to $15.

Advice

1. Make sure that you test early-morning urine. That's when the hormone is easiest to detect.

2. If you suspect that you might be pregnant and you get a negative result, repeat the test a week later. If the second result is negative and you still suspect pregnancy, or if you're still not menstruating, you should consult your doctor.

THE OVULATION PREDICTOR TEST

A woman is most fertile, and so most likely to become pregnant, during ovulation—the period during which an egg is released into the fallopian tubes.

The ovulation predictor test can predict ovulation up to three days in advance, and this makes it a valuable aid for women who have had difficulty conceiving. Couples who wish to plan their baby's birth for a particular time of the year can also benefit from these tests. The test depends on the presence of leutinizing hormone in the urine, which increases just prior to ovulation.

You should test your early-morning urine with the specially treated stick provided in the test kit. This has to be done once a day for about a week in midcycle. A change in color that correlates with the color guide included in the packet will tell you when you're ovulating.

Time   The results are usually clear within half an hour.

Cost   About $25.

Advice

1. Many things can interfere with conception. If you have trouble conceiving, make sure to consult an expert.

2. If you test positive for more than four days in a row, it could mean pregnancy, menopause, or an ovarian problem. In that case, make sure to consult your physician.

BLOOD IN THE STOOL

According to the American Cancer Society, three out of every four people with cancer of the large intestine could be saved if the condition were detected early enough. Since the presence of blood in the stool can be the first sign of intestinal cancer, and this blood is often not visible to the naked eye, the home test for stool blood could save your life. You must follow the instructions carefully, and take the results seriously. The American Cancer Society recommends this test for "screening" (for use by people who don't have symptoms) once a year after the age of 50.

Most of the home kits contain pads, tissues, or slides that change color when they come in contact with a stool sample that has blood in it.

Time   One to 15 minutes.

Cost $5 to $10.

Advice

1. The test is not a substitute for a rectal exam. The ACS recommends that you visit your doctor for a rectal exam once a year after the age of 40.

2. You must follow the instructions regarding diet and activity before using the kit. Exercise and ingestion of beef, vitamin C, horseradish, and aspirin can all produce false positive results. You wouldn't want to undergo a sigmoidoscopy just because you had steak for dinner.

3. There are two other things you should know about positive results before you use the test. Blood in the stool can be caused by other problems, such as an ulcer, or even something as simple as bleeding of the gums. Thus, this test can give "true positive" results, in the sense that they accurately record the presence of blood in the stool, without the blood being the result of colonic or rectal cancer. So don't become unduly alarmed if your stool tests positive.

   On the other hand, it is also possible for cancer to exist without any evidence of blood in the stool. So even if the test indicates that you have no blood in the stool, you should seek your doctor's advice if you have other symptoms or a family or personal history of the disease.

DIABETES

When the body's ability to metabolize sugar becomes impaired, the hallmark symptoms of diabetes appear: excessive thirst and urination, and fatigue.

One of the ways that doctors diagnose the disease is to check a patient's urine or blood for abnormally high levels of unmetabolized sugar. For years, diabetics have been using home kits that feature dipsticks to check for the presence of glucose in their urine. This same test is available to you, but it is best used by people who know they have diabetes to monitor treatment, rather than by nondiabetics as a diagnostic tool. You could have mild diabetes and miss it on a single urine test. Even for diabetics, the urine test is not as accurate as some doctors would like it to be, since the results can be affected by a bladder or kidney problem, or by the amount of fluid drunk during the day. For that reason, scientists have developed home kits for the monitoring of blood glucose levels in the diabetic. A spring-loaded device painlessly removes a spot of blood from your finger. You then touch the blood to a chemically treated strip, which you feed into an electronic machine.

This up-to-the-minute information on blood sugar levels helps the doctor and the patient make quick dietary and/or medication adjustments.

Time   Urine and blood: 1 to 2 minutes.

Cost   Urine tests: about $6.
Blood tests: about $18 to $20.
Electronic blood sugar meter: about $150.

Advice

1. Do not use either test for diagnosis. If you think you have diabetes, see your doctor for an evaluation.

2. If you are a diabetic and do use this home kit, have your doctor check you from time to time for the accuracy of your monitoring. Tight control of your blood sugar can make the difference between life and death.

URINARY TRACT INFECTION

Stubborn, recurrent bladder infections, called cystitis, are a familiar problem to many women. Now, when the telltale symptoms begin to appear—painful, burning urination and increased frequency—you can test your urine for infection.

One brand provides a dipstick that changes color in the presence of blood cells, another uses one that changes in the presence of nitrite-producing bacteria.

Test your urine on three straight mornings with a chemically treated strip. If it changes color, nitrite or blood cells are present.

Time   Less than 1 minute.

Cost   About $10.

Advice

1. Make sure at least to phone your doctor whenever you get symptoms of a urinary tract infection.

2. Ten percent of bacteria do not produce nitrite, so if you get a

negative result, and symptoms persist, make sure you see your doctor for a complete examination.

3. Never take an antibiotic without consulting your doctor.

IMPOTENCE

Impotence—the inability to get an erection—can be due to psychological or physical causes, or both.

This test makes use of the fact that men naturally have two to five erections per night while they sleep. A soft, cloth band that has three breakable plastic strips is wrapped around the penis before sleep. The strips will open whenever an erection occurs. If, upon awakening, all the plastic strips are broken, the cause is probably psychological. No breaks suggest a physical problem.

Time One night.

Cost $15 to $25.

Advice

1. Impotence can be a complex emotional and psychological problem. If you wish to use this as a preliminary test, do so. Whatever the results, make sure to seek the help of a professional. Many urologists have experience with the psychological aspects of impotence, both as cause and effect. If yours doesn't, and the cause turns out to be psychological, he should be able to refer you to someone who can help.

GONORRHEA

A man can now test for gonorrhea in the privacy of his home by collecting a sample of discharge from the urethra, the external opening on the penis, placing it on a slide, then mailing it to a lab for interpretation.

The test is not recommended for women, since they are less likely to have symptoms, and their anatomy is different. A pelvic exam is often necessary to detect gonorrhea in a woman.

For the man, the test is the same as the one used in the doctor's office. You can remain anonymous by using a code number, and you can choose to receive results by mail or telephone.

The makers of home tests for gonorrhea contend that a "personal" home test can help to control the spread of the disease because some men delay seeing a doctor out of embarrassment. Theoretically, it is a good idea. However, a false negative reading could lead to two serious problems:

● A falsely reassured patient might spread the gonorrhea infection further.

● Other venereal diseases may be the cause of the problem. They can produce similar symptoms and they may co-exist: we know that infection with one venereal disease may make you physically more susceptible to others. Since this test is gonorrhea-specific, it will miss the other STD's, and their spread might be similarly increased.

Time   A few days.

Cost $15 to $20.

Advice

1. If urinary discomfort or discharge remains despite a negative result from the lab, see a doctor. Avoid sexual contact until you can get medical treatment.

2. Inform any sexual partners of your symptoms.

Regarding STD's in general:

● If you have been diagnosed as having an STD, make sure your doctor checks for all the STD's. Remember, they often coexist, and you wouldn't want to miss them.

● You should be tested and treated if you have a partner who has been diagnosed as having an STD, even if you have no symptoms.

BLOOD PRESSURE

The home monitoring of blood pressure can mean the difference between life and death. It can lead to early detection, and it can help your doctor to monitor treatment.

You can purchase a stethoscope and blood pressure cuff at a medical supply store. Make sure the cuff fits. If it doesn't, it may give you an inaccurate reading. The standard cuff fits arms up to 13 inches in diameter, but there are larger cuffs for larger arms.

Follow the instructions in Chapter Three for the monitoring of blood pressure (page 44), and check Table One for healthy guidelines regarding what your blood pressure should be.

Time   Depends on experience; usually 2 to 5 minutes.

Cost $30 to $50 for a good stethoscope and blood pressure cuff.

Advice

1. High blood pressure rarely causes symptoms until it's too late. You can save your own life by learning how to monitor your blood

pressure. Even if you discover a high reading, take heart. Many people with high blood pressure can be treated with exercise and diet alone. Most of the rest respond well to medical treatment.

2. An average of three readings, taken five minutes apart, is more accurate than one reading.

3. Make sure a doctor or nurse checks your accuracy from time to time.

4. Exercise, stress, eating, or smoking can affect your blood pressure. Try to relax, and wait awhile after eating, exercising, or smoking before you do the test.

5. Good readings in someone who is being treated for high blood pressure are a reflection of successful treatment, not of cure. So, never stop your medication because you get good readings. The result could be a rebound elevation of your blood pressure, which could prove life-threatening.

GENDER CHOICE KITS: NOT THE RIGHT CHOICE

It used to be said that making love in the north wind produced a baby boy; the south wind, a baby girl. One manufacturer tried to make a mint on that type of advice—and got caught.

He produced a home-testing kit called Gender Choice, and sold it for $39.95. The kit contained diagrams and suggestions about timing, position, and type of sex, and a promise that you'd improve your chances of choosing your baby's sex by following the advice.

The fact is that your chances of having a baby girl are slightly greater than 50 percent, and conversely, for having a boy they are slightly less than 50 percent. No matter what you do. Genetics and personal medical history might make a difference, but the kit couldn't. When the FDA got wind of what the kit was promising, the packages were taken off the shelf, and the manufacturer was reprimanded.

The FDA acted quickly, but there were a few months when you could have wasted your money and had your hopes falsely elevated by the Gender Choice kit.

GENERAL GUIDELINES FOR USING HOME MEDICAL TESTS

False hopes might be the least of your problems if you use any of the other kits incorrectly or if you misinterpret their results.

In order to ensure your health and your peace of mind, follow the general guidelines below whenever you use a home medical testing kit:

1. *Follow the preparation instructions precisely.* Should you or shouldn't you eat? Are there any foods you must avoid before taking the test? If you're told not to eat, when should you have your last meal? Making a mistake on just one of these could affect the accuracy, comfort, and danger of the test.

   If medications need to be taken before the test, take them at the exact time you are instructed. Follow the instructions regarding rest and exercise as well.

2. *Follow the packaging and storage directions.* Heat, cold, dark, or light may affect a test's accuracy. Each test is different, so pack and store each kit exactly as directed.

3. *Check the expiration date.* An expired test is much more likely to yield inaccurate results. Don't take a chance. If yours has expired, get a new one.

4. *Read the instructions regarding the intent of the tests and its limitations carefully.* If you use a test for the wrong reason or if you don't understand its limitations, the effect could be worse than if you'd never done the test at all.

5. *Read the "How-To" instructions carefully.* If you collect a specimen, or time a test incorrectly, you could turn a negative into a positive, or vice versa.

6. *Read the instructions regarding interpretation carefully.* If you read a test incorrectly, you've wasted your time, and endangered yourself.

7. *If you're puzzled by the results, have the problem you tested for evaluated by your doctor.* These are only tests. They are capable of missing a diagnosis, or leading you down the wrong diagnostic path.

   All tests, whether they are performed in the home, the office, or hospital, sometimes need to be correlated with physical signs, history, and other tests in order to yield a correct diagnosis. In those cases, tests are meant to aid diagnostic workups, not replace them.

8. If you have any other questions at all about the test or the results, discuss them with your doctor or call the 800 number for product information that most manufacturers supply on the package insert.

9. If you suspect a test of misleading you, or the test's manufacturer of false advertising, call the United States Pharmacopia collect at 1-800-638-6725 (in Maryland, 301-881-0256.) You can write to this organization: Problem Reporting Program, 12601 Twinbrook Parkway, Rockville, MD 20852.

If you perform home tests properly, they are sure to improve your health care. They'll help you and your doctor to detect problems early, while there's still time for cure. They may even pick up a subtle disease before it causes symptoms and thus could mean the difference between life and death.

Use home tests to reduce the number of visits to your doctor's office. When you do have to see him, practice Smart Medicine by using the results of the tests and the rest of what you have learned to get the most out of your medical checkup.

1. *Give the most complete history possible.* Don't hold back. If you have a symptom, give the doctor every detail you can think of. When an ostrich sticks his head in the sand, the problem rarely goes away. In the case of medical diagnosis, the problem may get worse, since undiscovered illnesses can go on to become more serious problems.

2. *Report your own physical findings.* Tell your doctor how they may have changed since the symptoms first appeared, and how they compare to your "normal" medical exam, as described in Chapter Three.

3. *Do not walk into the doctor's office and announce your own diagnosis.* You'll want his well-trained mind to be objective.

4. *Once the exam is over, list the things you're worried about.* You may give the doctor a new idea, and at the very least you'll put your own mind at ease.

5. *When the doctor suggests other medical tests, ask our Six Crucial Questions and discuss all of the alternatives with him.*

6. *When the doctor suggests a diagnosis, ask what led to that conclusion.* You have a right to know, and a right to question the diagnosis and to participate in the decisions about treatment.

7. *When medicine is prescribed, make sure you understand all of the instructions, and all of the possible dangers and side effects.*

8. *Be insistent.* If the medicine doesn't work, if your symptoms don't go away, or if they change or worsen, insist on a repeat exam and further tests.

9. *Don't be afraid to ask questions.* If you're not satisfied with the answers, don't hesitate to seek a second opinion or to change doctors.

You can practice Smart Medicine every day—in your own home, at work, or at play. Your participation is crucial for the prevention and cure of disease. The information which you have obtained from this book will empower you with the knowledge and understanding to ensure that participation will be effective.

You have learned how to prevent medical mistakes, how to tell whether your doctor is competent, how to do your own physical exam to get the most out of your medical checkup, how to take medicines, and how to decide which medical tests you need. Use that knowledge to promote communication and develop a healthy partnership with your doctor.

You'll see him less often and have fewer medical tests, but each visit you do make and each test you do take will be more fruitful.

You'll save time and money while improving your chances of living a long, healthy life.

APPENDIX ONE
How to Choose a Good Doctor

Skip and Margo Greenway spent the first thirty-five years of their lives in a small town in Illinois. They got married, had two healthy children, and expected to grow old in the same town, tending the business that Skip had inherited from his father. But Skip got a job offer from a firm in Los Angeles, and the entire family decided to uproot themselves and move to a new home in the hills above Hollywood. They left their friends, the schools which the children had just started, and the doctor who had taken care of the entire family for the preceding five years.

The move went well and everyone made the adjustment to the faster pace and outdoor lifestyle of California. One night two years later, however, Chip developed severe chest pain. He didn't have a regular doctor, so Margo drove him to the nearest emergency room, where a diagnosis of severe angina pectoris, chest pain caused by insufficient blood flow to the heart, was made. Chip needed a thallium scan (see page 102) and an emergency angiogram (page 113). Margo became frightened and confused: "If I were home in Illinois," she thought, "Dr. Moseby would examine Skip, talk to the emergency doctor, and tell us what to do. He'd advise me about a second opinion and where to go for the tests. If only I'd taken the time to find a new doctor." She became even more distraught when, upon phoning home, she discovered that her oldest child, Charlie, had developed a fever of 104. She'd also neglected to find a doctor for the kids.

After two hours of frantic phone calls to relatives in Illinois, Margo sat down and discussed the entire problem with a chaplain and the head nurse at the hospital. They found a cardiologist for Skip, who had open heart surgery the next day. The babysitter brought the children by taxi to the emergency room, where the doctor on duty examined Charlie and diagnosed a middle ear infection. He prescribed antibiotics and referred Margo to a local pediatrician.

The whole family has since recovered, but Skip and Margo will never forget the excessive fear and confusion they went through simply because they hadn't bothered to find a new family doctor.

It sounds like a horror story, but unfortunately it's not uncommon. Millions of Americans don't have a regular doctor, and they're all vulnerable to the same type of near tragedy that befell Skip and Margo.

What would you do if you or a loved one developed chest pain, or one of your children developed a high fever and a rash? Would you go to the local emergency room and wait three hours to see a stranger? Would you let your fingers do the walking through the Yellow Pages in order to find an expert who could help you?

You might do either of those things, if you had to, but you wouldn't like it—you'd be frightened and worried.

If you're among those who do not have a regular doctor, or if you have decided that you need to change doctors, do you know how to go about choosing a good one?

If you already have a doctor whom you trust, what would you do if he became ill, retired, or moved away, or if *you* moved to a new town? Would you do what Margo did—neglect looking for a new doctor in the hope that your family would remain well and that you wouldn't need one?

EVERYONE NEEDS A REGULAR DOCTOR

A regular doctor is someone who knows you well, knows all of your idiosyncrasies and your complete medical history.

Someone whom you trust. Who can take care of you even if you are unable, because of illness, to communicate your medical history.

Someone who can save you time and anxiety during an emergency and, because he is so well acquainted with your health and medical history, stands the best chance of saving your life.

The time to learn how to choose a doctor is now, before an emergency occurs. The process is simple, and it can be broken down into five easy steps.

1. Decide what kind of doctor you need.
2. Make a list of the doctors in that specialty who are available in your area.
3. Narrow down the list by checking on the doctors' credentials, and the nature of their practices.
4. Interview the doctors on your final list.
5. Choose your regular doctor.

1. WHAT KIND OF DOCTOR DO YOU NEED?

Let's say you've moved to a new town and you've decided to find a doctor for your entire family. The first step in choosing the doctor will be to determine what your needs are. Should you choose a pediatrician, a family doctor, an internist, or a general practitioner?

Do you know the difference?

In order to decide what kind of doctor you need, and to find out how to choose one, you need to understand how doctors are trained, and what the designations mean.

How do doctors get their training, and what determines their specialty?

First, they get a medical doctorate, or "M.D." In the United States, medical doctors attend a medical school for four years. At the end of the second and fourth years, they are required to take a National Board Examination, which tests what they've learned. If they pass these exams and satisfactorily complete the requirements at their medical school, they receive their medical doctorate.

They can now call themselves "doctor," but they can't hang out a shingle and practice—yet. (The American Medical Association also recognizes D.O.'s—graduates of osteopathy school.)

Next, they do an internship. This is a one-year training program in a hospital setting, where M.D.'s actually take care of patients, under the supervision of residents (up until now, they've only studied patients and assisted in their treatment). This internship can be a rotating type, which includes medical, surgical, and other specialties, or can be strictly medical or surgical.

At the end of their internship year, they take a third set of National Boards, administered by the state where they plan to practice. If they pass (there's no guarantee that they will pass it the first time around), they receive a License to Practice General Medicine and Surgery in that state. (Many states offer reciprocal licenses.) Doctors who have been educated at foreign medical schools have to take an equivalency exam, either the ECFMG (Education Commission for Foreign Medical

Graduates) or FLEX (Foreign Student Licensing Exam), in order to get a United States license, and they may be required to repeat their internship. Once they complete their internships and pass these exams, they can obtain a license and open a practice.

If they take no further formal residency training (see below), they become general practitioners—G.P.'s. In the old days, most doctors were G.P.'s. There are fewer now, but they still exist, and many who keep up with the current medical literature are considered to be highly competent as general physicians.

If they elect to continue their education and become specialists, they choose a residency in a particular field, which consists of two or more years of more advanced training, during which they care for patients and supervise interns in a hospital. At the end of their residency, they must take a test in their specialty administered by the Board in order to be board-certified. Unlike internship and licensure, board certification is not required by law; doctors do not have to be board-certified to call themselves a particular type of specialist.

It's always a good idea to ask someone who claims he's a specialist whether or not he's board-certified.

If you do not choose a general practitioner as your primary-care physician, you may choose someone who has done a residency and is board-certified in one of the two following specialties:

Family Practice

Family practice doctors take training in pediatrics, general family medicine, general surgery, psychiatry, obstetrics, gynecology, and emergency medicine. They have a wide breadth of experience but less intensive training in each field than do the respective specialists of those fields.

Internal Medicine

The internist takes advanced training in the treatment of medical problems that occur in adults. Within this field there are also many subspecialties, including cardiology (the treatment of heart disease) and oncology (the treatment of cancer).

After the choice of your primary-care physician, you and your family may also require the services of a doctor who is board-certified in one of the following specialties:

Pediatrics

Pediatrics is the care of children, from birth until the teenage years. Some pediatricians care for the same patients into their twenties, but they are not as qualified as family practitioners or internists to care for adults.

There are many subspecialties within pediatrics, including pediatric surgery and pediatric psychiatry. As with all subspecialties, they require additional years of training after residency.

Obstetrics and Gynecology

These specialties deal with the medical and surgical care of the pregnant and nonpregnant woman, and the delivery of babies. Because of the wide variety of health issues specific to females, many women use their gynecologist as their only regular doctor. This may suffice for many problems, but obstetricians and gynecologists are not fully trained in the treatment of all adult diseases. A gynecologist should no more be a woman's only primary-care physician than a urologist should be a man's.

General Surgery

A residency in general surgery can lead to a specialty in the treatment of a wide variety of surgical problems. More specialized treatment may require a fellowship in a subspecialty such as plastic surgery, head and neck surgery, thoracic (chest and heart) surgery, or neurosurgery.

Finally, you may on occasion and for specific problems require the help of someone trained in the following specialties:

Anesthesiology

Anesthesiologists are trained in the administration of anesthesia. They function most often in the operating room.

Dermatology

The medical and surgical care of the skin.

Emergency Medicine

This is one of the newer fields in medicine. Emergency physicians are now full-time doctors trained in the care of medical and surgical emergencies, from heart attacks to gunshot wounds. They are not trained in chronic care, but have their own residency, and their own certifying board.

Ophthalmology

The medical and surgical care of the eye.

Psychiatry

A medical doctor who completes a medical or rotating internship, then takes advanced training in the treatment of psychiatric disorders.

Radiology

Radiologists complete their internship, then take specialty training in the reading of x-rays and other diagnostic procedures, such as ultrasound and CAT scans. They can take advanced training in radiotherapy, the administration of radiation treatments to cancer patients, or invasive radiology—the performance of such procedures as angiograms.

Urology

The medical and surgical treatment of male and female urinary tract disorders, including disorders of the genitals, bladder, prostate, and kidneys.

It can get confusing, but you can make it easy. Find out which specialties are available in your area—this by itself may help you narrow your choices. If it doesn't, take it step by step:

You may need a pediatrician or a family practitioner for your children, and the women in the family will need an obstetrician-gynecologist.

If you can, you should choose an internist, a family practitioner, or a general practitioner as your primary-care physician.

If the differences in the training don't help limit your choice, don't worry. Include all three types on your list. You'll decide once you meet them.

Now, on to the search.

2. MAKE A LIST

Once you've decided on the type of doctor you need (or even if you haven't yet completely narrowed it down), make a list of candidates in your area.

- Call your local emergency room or hospital, most of them have doctors listed by specialty. Some have full-time referral services. There are even some medical referral services springing up in shopping centers.
- If you are changing doctors because you have moved and are still in contact with your old doctor, ask him if he knows or can suggest anyone.
- Ask your friends for suggestions.
- Call your local medical society; not all doctors belong, but it's a good source of referrals.
- Look in the Yellow Pages (now, not later).
- Look in the *American Medical Association Directory of Physicians*. It's available in most local libraries.

You may not need all of these sources, but you should be able to compile a pretty long list by using some of them.

3. NARROW DOWN YOUR LIST BY CHECKING ON THE DOCTOR'S CREDENTIALS AND THE NATURE OF HIS PRACTICE

- Consider the location of his office and the hospitals he practices in. Are they close by and convenient?
- Call to ask about his office hours and insurance policies. Do they meet your needs?
- Call the local medical society and see if he is a member and if any disciplinary action has ever been taken against him. Membership doesn't ensure competence, and you can't be sure about the nature of disciplinary charges, but these pieces of information may help.
- Call the state board of medical quality assurance in your state and make sure he has a current license, and ask the same questions regarding disciplinary actions as you did of the local medical society.
- Ask his patients, and other doctors, if you know any, about his reputation.

By this time, your list will have shrunk to reasonable size.

4. INSPECT THE OFFICES AND INTERVIEW THE DOCTORS WHO ARE STILL ON YOUR LIST

You have the right and the need to know everything you can about your doctor's practice, competency, and demeanor. Remember, you are not auditioning to be someone's patient, the doctor is being interviewed for a job.

The questions you ask, and the answers you receive (in terms of both content and attitude) will help you to make your final decision. When you first enter the office, ask yourself the following questions:

- Is the office clean and well organized?
- Are the office personnel and the nurses courteous and friendly, or abrupt and uncommunicative?

You won't be charged just for looking around, and you may be able to scratch some doctors off the list before you ever reach them.

The Doctor's Education and Training

Explain to one of the office personnel that you want to get all the information you can before choosing a doctor, and that you'd like to ask some questions about the doctor's education, training, and practice. You have a right to this information. If you can't get straight answers, don't hesitate to shop somewhere else.

When you consider the nature of a doctor's education, don't expect to make your choice solely on the basis of his credentials. Other factors will be equally important.

However, the quality and extent of the education may play a critical role in your final decision.

- *Where did he go to medical school?*
  It doesn't so much matter whether the doctor went to Harvard or Howard, as much as it matters that he went to an accredited school, and that the course of study was completed.
- *Where did he do an internship?*
  As with medical schools, most hospitals provide good training. But make sure that the medical school is accredited and that the internship was completed.
- *Is he licensed?*
  Make sure. And ask if the license has ever been revoked or suspended.

- *Did he do a residency?*
  If so, where?
- *What is his specialty?*
- *Is he board-certified in that specialty?*
- *If not, has he taken the test?*

  Now we're getting to the substance. You'll get to know much more about the doctor's specific training. Keep in mind that board certification is not the sine-qua-non of competency; some good doctors fail the test, and some that pass never keep up with their education. If you like a doctor, and are convinced of his competency, the lack of board certification should not completely rule him out, just as its presence should not prompt you to choose someone you don't like. However, if you're on the fence, it can help you to decide.

- Does the doctor have a subspecialty?

  This may help if you have a particular chronic problem. A cardiologist may be best for someone with heart disease, for instance. Or a rheumatologist, who treats bones and joints medically, might be most helpful for someone with arthritis.

The Doctor's Practice

You will want to inform yourself of some practical aspects of the doctor's practice, to make sure he can give you the kind of service you need, taking into consideration your family makeup, finances, and schedule, for example. You will want to ask some or all of the following questions:

- *What are the office hours and the policies regarding insurance?*
- *Is lab work done in the office, or is it sent out?* Some doctors do their own, which could save you time and money. If this is the case, ask whether the lab technicians are certified by a laboratory licensing board. You wouldn't want to save money but get inaccurate lab results. If the work is sent out, you have a right to know which laboratory it's sent to, and whether or not that lab is certified. A few years ago a number of inaccurate lab results were reported on Pap smears, and it led to quite a controversy.
- *Who covers for the doctor when he's off?* If you don't know who covers when he's ill, off duty, or out of town, you'll only have investigated part of his practice. You need to know whether his partner or associate is as skilled as he is, and whether their demeanor and communicativeness are similar.
- *What is the policy about phone calls and emergencies?* This can make all the difference in the world. Many doctors provide special hours for phone

calls. Some, such as pediatricians, have special help to answer them. Although many doctors handle their patients' emergencies themselves, some never take emergency calls after hours. You'll want to know the answers ahead of time.

● *Does the doctor teach?* As with medical society membership and board certification, the answer to this question won't give you an absolute definition of his competence. But it takes an interested, committed doctor to teach, and, if he does, he's more likely to be up on the latest changes in medical care.

Once you've finished questioning the office personnel, you'll want to talk to the doctor as well. In an ideal world, you'd be able to do this without cost, but in reality, you'll probably only succeed once you've made your first appointment with the doctor—which may cost you a small fee. In either case, however, don't fail to ask him the following questions, and don't hesitate to seek a different doctor if the answers are unsatisfactory.

● *What is your attitude toward second opinions?*
The answer will speak volumes about the doctor's nature. If he becomes defensive and uptight, he may just be having a bad day (ask him—he has a right to one every once in a while), or his attitude may be suggestive of just the type of doctor you want to avoid. If, on the other hand, he's open and forthright, you've taken a step in the right direction.
● *What is your attitude toward home medical tests, and toward my participation in my own medical care in general?*
This could be the clincher. He doesn't have to give a wholesale endorsement of home medical tests—they do have their limitations (see Chapter Seventeen), but he should be anxious to have you participate in your own health care. It can help him to prevent and treat disease, while ensuring your health. In today's world, medical diagnosis and treatment work best as a partnership.
You're reading this book because you want to participate. It will help if your doctor is of the same mind. If he's not, then you don't want him as your doctor.

5. CHOOSE YOUR REGULAR DOCTOR

By now, you should have fairly complete pictures of all the doctors on your final list. The substance and the nature of their answers should have told you a lot about them, and about their practices.

Think about it, but don't make your decision immediately. Cross the doctors who didn't fill the bill off your list. Then sleep on it.

Review the doctors whom you are still considering, and remember your conversations with them. Did they use "doctorese," that strange medical language known only to physicians? Were they unwilling—or unable—to take the time to explain things slowly, in plain English? Did they encourage your involvement in medical diagnosis and treatment?

When you consider all the factors—your needs and the doctor's practice, competence, and personality—you'll have your answer. Once you've chosen your regular doctor, you'll have one more crucial thing to do.

GET TO KNOW YOUR DOCTOR OVER THE COURSE OF TIME AND CONSTANTLY REASSESS WHETHER OR NOT YOU WANT TO STAY WITH HIM

You'll learn much more than you could have during the initial interview, and things can change—for the better or worse. You should remain open and flexible, and willing to reconsider on the basis of your new knowledge. Ask yourself the following questions:

- Has he lived up to your expectations? Did his answers reflect what really goes on?
- Has he remained communicative and accessible to you? Or is he now hard to reach and less available?
- Has his coverage, office time, and follow-up been what you hoped it would be?
- Does he remain open to your participation in your own health care, and to occasional second opinions?

If changes have occurred for the worse, or you've noticed some of the signs of incompetence (see Chapter Two), you've got to be willing to reconsider, and change doctors if necessary.

Your life may depend on it.

APPENDIX TWO
How to Choose Your Medical Insurance

I first met a girl we'll call Carrie Wessler at three A.M. on a dark, rainy night when she was brought to our emergency room by ambulance after being in a bad car accident.

Carrie was awake—and frightened. She was only 19 years old, and her parents were out of town for the weekend. The accident had occurred while she was on her way home from a party, and it wasn't her fault. A drunk driver had suddenly swerved into her lane and hit her car, forcing it into the center divider. Considering the circumstances, she was lucky: her only injury was a deep wound in her right leg. But she had already lost nearly two quarts of blood.

And the worst news was yet to come.

X-rays revealed that she had shattered both of the bones in the lower leg, and a close examination made me suspect that a piece of bone had cut right through the leg's most important artery. She needed major surgery—and fast.

We began a blood transfusion and notified the orthopedic and vascular surgeons on call, but when I told them that Carrie had no proof of medical insurance, they refused to come in.

"She's sure she has coverage," I said; "her father owns the largest industrial company in town, and the family lives in one of the most affluent neighborhoods in Los Angeles."

But the surgeons insisted that they were only following hospital policy; years of treating uninsured patients who either could not or would not pay their bills had forced the hospital into debt, and the administration had decided to take a hard line. They insisted on the transfer of all patients without proof of insurance to the County Hospital—unless they were in life or limb-threatening danger.

I argued that Carrie *was* in a limb-threatening danger; if the broken bone had severed the artery, she would lose her leg.

The surgeons asked me to repeat her blood count (to see how much blood had been lost) and her examination, have the emergency room clerk do everything she could to locate Carrie's parents, then call them back.

By the time we knew the results of the second blood test, we still had not found her parents. But more than an hour had passed, and the leg was looking worse. The surgeons finally consented to come in.

The operation took four hours, and they saved Carrie's leg. Three operations and two years later, she's walking without a limp. As it turned out, however, she had no insurance. She owes the doctors and the hospital nearly $50,000.

Her story, unfortunately, is not unique. Millions of Americans have no medical insurance, and only 10 percent of those people cite financial problems as their reason.

Carrie's father explained that he had been unhappy about the state of medical care in this country, and that he objected to rising insurance costs. He hoped his healthy family wouldn't need medical care, and he believed that the savings would be worth the risk.

He may have been right about our medical system; many people feel that it could use a drastic overhaul, but he couldn't have been more wrong about the risk.

You can't afford to let this sort of thing happen to you. No matter how you feel about the cost and delivery of medical care in this country, you have to face the facts.

- Illness and injury can strike at any time.
- Until the system changes, good medical insurance is the only way to protect your health, your peace of mind, and your pocketbook.

There are many different types of medical insurance available, and the difficulty in choosing among them may be one of the reasons that people delay getting coverage. But if you examine your own needs carefully and consider the advantages and disadvantages of each plan, you should be able to find one that is right, and affordable, for you.

WHAT DO YOU NEED?

Everyone's medical needs are different—they depend on age, sex, and personal and family medical history.

But some aspects of coverage are always essential:

Hospitalization Insurance

"Hospitalization" covers the costs of your room, food, lab tests, medicines, operations, and doctors' bills while you're in the hospital. Every plan is different, and you should find out the answers to the following questions ahead of time:

- Does the policy pay from my first day of hospitalization? Some don't, and you may end up paying a lot more out of your pocket than you expected to—if you don't read the fine print.
- What doesn't it include? Are there restrictions on medicines, type of hospitalizations (for example, are hospital costs related to pregnancy and delivery), doctors bills, or operations. Does it specify private, semiprivate or ward bed?
- How much is paid for at the outset? One hundred percent, or 80 percent? Is there a deductible—some amount you have to pay before the insurance company starts paying? It could be as much as $1,000.
- How much is paid each day? Do you only get a certain amount, like $100 for every day you're in the hospital? If you don't ask now, you could be in trouble later on.
- Is there a limit on length of stay? Do payments stop after a certain dollar amount of bills or number of days?
- Does the policy cover all hospitals, and all doctors, or only certain ones?

Major Medical Insurance

The "major medical" part of your insurance covers you for medical costs other than those covered by your hospital coverage, such as doctor's fees, physical therapy, the cost of x-rays, blood tests, other diagnostic procedures and treatments, but it may not cover everything.

Ask the following questions:

- What, if any, is the deductible? How much must you pay before the insurance company starts paying?
- What is the most the insurance company will pay, $20,000 or $2

million? There is wide variation, and the answer could leave you penniless if you don't find out ahead of time.

- Will you have to pay part of the costs? This is called a co-payment.
- What else does the major medical provide? Does it cover care in the home? Does it cover specialty care, like physical therapy for an injury? Does it cover dental care and/or maternity care? Many regular policies do not cover these. Make sure you ask.
- What doesn't the major medical provide? Some policies predetermine the types of things that they consider appropriate in medical diagnosis and treatment—and the things they consider inappropriate. They usually have a list of these, so it's a good idea to look at it ahead of time. Whenever a test or treatment is planned, work with your doctor. Ask him whether it will be covered by your insurance.
- What about emergency care? Are there any restrictions? In the case of set-fee health plans or health maintenance organizations (see below) and some restricted private insurance plans, you may need approval before you receive emergency treatment away from the home hospital. If you don't get it, the money could come out of your own pocket.
- What about preventive medicine? There is a lot of variation in this. Beware! With all of our interest in preventive care, many people get regular checkups, blood tests, and other types of preventive care that insurance companies may not cover. Check before you buy coverage, and check again with your insurance company before you have any preventive work done.

Catastrophic Insurance

"Catastrophic" refers to coverage other than hospitalization and major medical insurance—it covers you in the event of a debilitating, expensive, long-term illness. It is not automatically part of every policy, and may cost more, but it can mean the difference between poverty and comfort if a long-term, catastrophic illness or injury strikes.

Other Possible Needs

- **Nursing home care.** Most regular policies don't cover this, so you may want to ask. If you're interested, you may have to get a separate policy.
- **Elderly coverage.** You've probably seen a lot of TV commercials for insurance plans offering extra care for the elderly. Many people need it. Medicare does not cover all problems, and Medicare payments may be very restricted. On the other hand, you should be aware that a recent study published in the *New England Journal of Med-*

icine showed that people over the age of 65 had more and better medical insurance than any other age group. Beware of overspending as well as of being underinsured.

- **Maternity care.** If your regular policy doesn't have it, you may not be able to get it after you become pregnant.
- **Dental care.** Many plans exclude dental coverage, and many others pay only part of the cost.
- **Hospice care.** This coverage is for people with chronic or terminal illnesses.
- **Home health care.** This will protect people with chronic, debilitating illnesses, or injuries and problems that require home rehabilitation, such as stroke or physical injury from an accident.

TYPES OF INSURANCE PLANS

Once you've decided what your insurance needs are, you can choose the plan that best suits you. There are many different types of policies and plans, but they generally fall into one of three categories.

Conventional or Private Insurance

Private plans usually cost the most and give you the widest choice—of doctors, treatments, and hospitals. They come in two basic forms.

NO-RESTRICTIONS PLAN   "No-restriction insurance" may seem a bit misleading. There will still be some restrictions on coverage (ask the questions above to make sure that there are no surprises), but the policy does not restrict you to certain doctors or hospitals.

PREFERRED-PROVIDER PLAN A "conventional" insurance company can offer this variation on their own policy, which costs less than their "no-restriction" policy, but offers fewer choices. The insurance company gives you a list of doctors, hospitals, and other services with whom it contracts, where they will pay a higher percentage of the cost than if you go to someone with whom they have no contract.

Preferred-Provider Organizations

Preferred-provider organizations (PPO's) are a cross between the "conventional" type and the health maintenance organization (HMO) (see below).

A PPO is a group of tightly bound doctors who contract to provide service together. The costs (and choices) may be a bit less than with completely private insurance, and a bit more than with an HMO.

Health Maintenance Organizations

An HMO provides you with all your medical care, for a fixed sum. Some HMO's require you to pay a minor "co-payment," but the total cost is usually less than with conventional insurance.

There are many different types of HMO's. Some are housed in one building, or one hospital. Others have a number of clinics, hospitals, and doctors within a short distance of one another. Some contract with a group of independent physicians who still treat private patients, as well. If you elect an HMO with this type of plan, you'll go to doctors' private offices, but be otherwise bound by the rules and restrictions of the HMO. Some others offer only general care; they're not associated with a hospital. If the need for hospitalization arises, they pay the costs, but only if they approve the hospital and the physician taking care of you.

In one way or another, the HMO will cover your major medical and hospitalization bills. But you'll still need to ask all of the same questions regarding coverage and restrictions that you would ask if you were selecting conventional insurance.

THE ADVANTAGES AND DISADVANTAGES OF EACH TYPE OF PLAN

Conventional Insurance

ADVANTAGES
1. Wide, unrestricted choice in doctors, hospitals, location and type of care. With the preferred-provider variation, the cost may be less but the choices may be more limited. In either case, be sure you ask all the questions about coverage, and find out exactly what's included and what isn't.
2. If you already have a doctor you like, you can stay with him if you choose private insurance. He or an associate may be reachable twenty-four hours a day, seven days a week. With PPO's or HMO's, the doctors' availability may be more limited.
3. Emergency care will be paid for, no matter what hospital you go to or are taken to.
4. Some people argue that higher-cost private insurance makes it more likely that your doctor will be of higher quality. Others say it means only that they will charge more and do more tests.

DISADVANTAGES

1. The costs are higher. Not only does the policy cost more, but other costs, such as prescriptions, may not be covered.
2. There is less continuity of care among doctors. Private doctors may not communicate with each other as much as those within the same HMO do, and communication could be important if you need more than one type of care. This disadvantage may be overcome with a good primary-care doctor and a lot of effort on your part. But it's usually simpler in an HMO, where your records are always available to all consulting medical specialists.
3. There is less peer review. Private physicians may not check on each other's policies and practices as much as they do in an HMO. But there are regular reviews of private physicians by licensing boards and quality assurance groups. And you can do your own quality assurance by reading Chapters 2 and 3.

HMO's

ADVANTAGES

1. Costs are lower. The policy will probably be less expensive than conventional insurance. Also, many allied services and ancillary costs, such as medicines, may be included in your set fee.
2. An HMO is convenient, because all of your medical services are in one place. Note that this may be a disadvantage if you live far from the HMO.
3. Preventive-medicine checkups will usually be paid for. Private insurance may not cover them.
4. There is more peer review. There may be more internal reviews of the quality of care than there would be in a private setting.
5. A possible advantage is better continuity in care. When you get all of your medical care in one facility or within one geographical area, you may have easier access to different specialties, and your doctors may have easier access to your medical charts and to one another.

DISADVANTAGES

1. There is less choice in doctors and other services; you have to use those within the HMO. Keep in mind though, that within the HMO there may be a wide variety available, and you may be able to choose your own primary-care doctor.
2. If you already have a private doctor whom you like, you may have to change to an HMO doctor.
3. Emergency care may be problematical. If you can't make it to the HMO, you may need phone approval before emergency care at other

hospitals will be paid for. With some HMO's, you may have to pay first, then try to bill them later.

Even if you make it to the HMO, your primary-care physician may not be reachable twenty-four hours a day, or seven days a week.

4. Some people argue that set fees make it less likely that HMO doctors will be of high quality. Others say that HMO doctors have more time for you because they are not as competitive as private doctors and provide better care.

MAKING THE CHOICE

Your choice of medical insurance should be based on your individual lifestyle, economic situation, and medical needs.

1. Make a List of All Your Medical Needs.

2. Decide on Your Priorities.

Ask yourself the following questions:

- *What coverage do you need?* Use the descriptions and questions at the beginning of this chapter as your guidelines.
- *What's most important to you?* For instance, is free choice of physician more important than low cost? Is unrestricted emergency care more important than free preventive checkups?
- *How much are you willing to pay for insurance?*
- *How much wouldn't you mind paying out of pocket if you found yourself in need of medical care?* Your answer here should be tempered with the knowledge of your own medical and family history, which makes certain illnesses more or less likely. Don't make the assumption that everyone will remain healthy. Plan for the worst, so that your coverage will be the best. This doesn't mean that everyone needs catastrophic insurance. That's an individual decision, based on needs and economics.

3. Consider the Advantages and Disadvantages of Each Plan, and Decide Which Plan Best Suits Your Needs.

Which yields the best combination of convenience, safety, coverage, cost and peace of mind?

4. If You're Still Unsure, Ask to Interview the Doctors and Medical Specialists Who Work Within Each Plan.

For conventional insurance this may not be necessary, since your choice of doctor may be unrestricted, but it will be necessary if you're trying to decide among conventional insurance, a PPO, and an HMO, or among several different HMOs. Use the guidelines for choosing a doctor outlined in Chapter Two. Once you've completed the interviews and considered your own needs, you should have your answer, and know which medical insurance plan you want to subscribe to.

Whatever you do, don't delay the decision. You wouldn't want to be in Carrie's shoes tomorrow. If you become unhappy with the plan you selected, don't panic; there's always time to change.

APPENDIX THREE
How to Choose a Hospital and an Emergency Room

No one likes to be hospitalized; it can be a frightening, depressing experience. Sometimes, however, it's necessary, and it can be even more frightening if you aren't sure you've selected the best hospital.

Consider the following two scenarios.

Your spouse develops chest pain and is taken by ambulance to the local hospital. After a few days and a lengthy workup, the hospital cardiologist tells you that a coronary bypass operation will be needed. Your mate's life is not in immediate danger, but the operation should be done within the next few weeks.

Do you stay in this hospital, or investigate others? Do you go to a teaching hospital, or to a private hospital. Do you know the difference?

Your best friend calls you in a panic: her doctor discovered a lump under her arm that has to be removed. He thinks it's benign but he's not sure and doesn't want to wait. He has suggested your friend be admitted to the hospital in the morning. Compounding her anxiety, he has given her a choice between two hospitals. One is a world-renowned university hospital where she's afraid that she'll get "poked and handled by a bunch of medical students and interns." The other has a "country-club" reputation, with good food and nice paintings, but she's concerned about the care she'd receive in the event of a complication or an emergency.

Can you help her decide?

Situations like these occur all the time. In some cases, the answer is simple: you go where your doctor is on staff.

It's more difficult when you have a choice, or if your doctor doesn't specialize in the problem you need taken care of, or if you don't have a private doctor.

Do you know what the different types of hospitals are? Would you be able to decide which hospital is best for you? Most of us hope that we'll never have to make that decision, but the need for hospitalization often occurs without warning. You'll ensure both your health and your peace of mind if you learn how to choose ahead of time.

TYPES OF HOSPITALS

For our purposes, the most important distinctions are in services offered, quality of care, the presence or absence of teaching facilities, and the nature of the accommodations.

On the basis of those criteria, our definitions may be a bit different than what you might hear if you asked a hospital administrator to define the type of hospital that he runs.

The Private, Non-University-Affiliated Hospital

This is just what the name says. It is owned, administered, and funded privately. The owners may be doctors, private individuals, a religious organization, or a corporation that owns many hospitals. The facility will be staffed by private physicians and allied health-care personnel, and there will be no residents or interns on duty. It may specialize in one, two, or many types of care (such as pregnancy, or heart disease), but in most cases it is a "primary- and secondary-care facility." This means it gets referrals from its own emergency room, private citizens, and doctors. It rarely gets "tertiary referrals," patients who have complicated medical problems that the staffs of other hospitals have been unable to handle.

ADVANTAGES
1. Accommodations may be more pleasant than in a public hospital.
2. Care may be more personal.
3. You will not be touched or examined by anyone other than your own physicians, nurses, and technicians.

DISADVANTAGES
1. In the event of an emergency or complication, expert medical care may have to be called in. Nurses are present around the clock, but

doctors may not be. For your piece of mind, before you check in ask whether or not an emergency doctor is always in the hospital.
2. Being a primary- and secondary-care facility, it may not have the facilities to diagnose and treat more complex problems.

The Medical School–Affiliated Private Hospital

This hospital is run in much the same way as a purely private hospital with the exception that medical students, interns and/or residents are present to help provide medical care.

ADVANTAGES
1. Accommodations and care may be as personal as in a nonaffiliated private hospital.
2. Having a medical school affiliation may encourage teaching among the private physicians, which may improve their ability to care for more complex problems.
3. There may be doctors on duty more often than with the nonaffiliated hospital.

DISADVANTAGES
1. You may be subjected to more tests, more examinations, and more probing hands than you would otherwise be. Most hospitals allow you to refuse examinations by anyone other than your own doctor, but there may be a natural tendency to order more tests in these facilities, to give medical students and technicians practice in administering and interpreting them.

The University Hospital

This type of hospital is housed on the grounds of a university or medical school, and has medical students, interns, and residents in attendance. If he works here, your private doctor will also be on the teaching staff of the medical school and/or hospital.

ADVANTAGES
1. In many cases, university hospitals are "tertiary-care facilities": they handle patients with medical problems other hospitals can't handle, as well as regular patients. Their ability to deal with complex diagnostic dilemmas may be superior to that of private hospitals.
2. Residents and interns are on duty twenty-four hours a day, seven days a week.
3. Teaching ability is at a premium, so the average physician in this

hospital may be more up-to-date on new and complex procedures than is the average physician in a private hospital.

This does not imply that every university-hospital doctor is better educated than every private-hospital doctor. Many private doctors teach at medical schools and in universities, and no amount of university schooling can guarantee quality of care.

DISADVANTAGES
1. Accommodations may not be as comfortable as in purely private hospitals, although they may be more pleasant than some publicly owned facilities.
2. You may be poked, handled, and tested more often. Again, you can refuse, but there's that natural tendency toward more testing.

The Public Hospital

This institution may be owned by the city, state, or county. It may also be a veterans' hospital—not technically public because it's limited to veterans, but owned by the federal government.

ADVANTAGES
1. Costs are lower, because the public agency handles at least part of the cost, and you pay only what it is determined you can afford.
2. Many public hospitals are affiliated with medical schools and so are staffed by residents, interns, and attending staff physicians, who also teach medicine. In that case, public hospitals have many of the advantages of the medical school– and university-affiliated hospitals: teaching, and around-the-clock doctors.

DISADVANTAGES
1. Accommodations may not be as pleasant as in a private hospital.
2. Public hospitals affiliated with university or medical schools have the same disadvantages: less privacy and more tests.

The Specialty Hospital

This term refers only to hospitals created to specialize in a single area of medical treatment; examples are cancer hospitals, hospices, or rehabilitation facilities.

ADVANTAGE   Singularity of care and purpose mean that staff in these hospitals will know the most about the area, and available medical services and the physical plant will most likely also reflect this specialization.

DISADVANTAGE   A specialty hospital may be unable to handle some other medical problems outside of its specialty area. Before electing this type of hospital, make sure that it is at least equipped to deal with emergencies and complications.

HOW DO YOU DECIDE?

The choice of hospital is an individual one and depends on your medical needs and your personal priorities. You can make the decision simple by considering the following factors:

1. *Where is your doctor on staff?* If you prefer to be with your own doctor, this may be the only question you need to ask—as long as your insurance plan covers you at that hospital, and it has the facilities you need.
2. *What does your doctor recommend?* If your doctor is not on staff where you need specialized care, or if other factors, such as location and insurance, cause you to consider hospitals other than the ones where your doctor practices, he may be able to help. He may know a specialist at another hospital whom he feels is qualified to treat you.
3. *What does your insurance pay for, and what can you afford?* Wherever you choose to be hospitalized, make sure *ahead of time* that your insurance will cover you at that facility.

    If you belong to an HMO, you may have no choice of facility, unless you wish to pay on your own.

    Your choices may also be limited if you belong to a preferred payment plan.
4. *What sort of problem are you being hospitalized for?* Certain hospitals are known for their obstetrical departments, others for their cardiac-care units. You may want to consider the hospital's reputation for treating your specific problem before you make your final decision.
5. *How likely is it that you'll need emergency care or treatment of a complex problem (tertiary care) while in the hospital?*

    If the need for emergency or tertiary care seems likely, or if you simply prefer around-the-clock doctor care you may want to choose a university- or medical school–affiliated hospital. Twenty-four-hour nursing care can be purchased at any hospital.
6. *How important to you are accommodations?*

    If all other things are equal, the type of accommodations, in terms of environment, privacy, comfort, and food, may help you decide.
7. If you've narrowed it down, but the first six considerations have not led to a final decision, investigate each hospital further. You won't be

able to do this in an emergency, so take the time to do it before an emergency occurs.

- Do an on-site inspection. Take a firsthand look at the advantages and disadvantages of each hospital.
- Talk to doctors and people who work at each hospital, and to patients who have been hospitalized there. Find out their impressions about the quality and nature of care.
- Check on the rating and record of each hospital. Call or write your local or state health department. They should be able to give you the results of the hospital's review by the Joint Council for Accreditation of Hospitals (JCAH), which routinely inspects and evaluates each hospital, and tell you if the hospital has ever been cited or punished for health or medical violations.

Once you've considered all of these factors, you should have your hospital picked out.

If more than one fits the bill, don't fret. The steps you've taken will ensure your safety and comfort at any one of them.

When you do check in, take a few final precautions to make sure that it turns out that way:

1. Read the admission papers carefully. These will tell you what's expected of you in terms of payment and behavior, so that you do not infringe on other patients. They will also explain visiting policy and other hospital protocol, including your rights.
2. Read all consent forms before signing them.
3. Realize that you can leave the hospital any time you wish. Your doctor may advise otherwise, and you may have to "sign out against medical advice" ("a.m.a."). Although I don't advise doing this unless your care has been so unsatisfactory or your outside needs are so pressing that it becomes unavoidable, it is your right. You are not a prisoner.
4. Insist on privacy. Your medical situation should never be discussed where other patients can hear or with any other people unless you give permission, and you should never be examined without having the doors closed or the curtains drawn.
5. If you are unhappy with any aspect of your medical care, or you witness the mistreatment of any other patient, call the department of health and report it. This is the type of information that you yourself may have sought when you were choosing a hospital. Your report might result in corrective action and it could help to ensure someone else's safety, comfort, and peace of mind.

CHOOSING AN EMERGENCY ROOM

Many emergency rooms operate on a contract basis: they provide emergency service for hospitals but they have their own staff and their own administration. This means that it's possible (albeit unlikely) for a poorly run emergency room to be housed in a good hospital, or vice versa. In any case your choice of emergency rooms may be different than your choice of hospitals.

If your problem is life-threatening and you're transported by city or county ambulance, you won't have a choice—you'll be taken to the closest hospital. In all other emergencies, such as cuts, allergic reactions, or infections, you'll have to decide on your own. As with your choice of hospital, you should get to know the emergency rooms in your area before the problem occurs, so you won't have to make the decision at the last minute.

1. Consider the location of the emergency room. Drive to each one at different times of the day to find out which is easiest and quickest to reach. This information could make the difference between life and death if a severe emergency occurs.
2. Call and ask what each emergency room's "designation" is. There are three types of emergency room.
   - "Stand-by" emergency rooms may be open or have a doctor in attendance only part time; they may accept only "walk-in patients" and no emergency paramedic ambulances.
   - "Full basic" emergency rooms have a physician on duty twenty-four hours a day who is skilled in emergency care. They accept all ambulances and all emergencies.
   - "Trauma centers" offer all of the same services as a "full basic" emergency room. In addition, they have a complete surgical team on duty. This means that they can usually perform major "trauma" surgery on patients who have life-threatening injuries more quickly and, in some cases, more expertly than other emergency rooms.

     In all other ways, trauma centers offer no advantage over "full basic" emergency rooms for the treatment of other types of emergencies such as heart attacks, cuts, or asthmatic attacks.
3. Ask neighbors and your doctor about the quality of care each emergency room offers.
4. Call and ask the emergency room clerks what they require for payment. Some accept credit cards and checks, and some will simply bill you or your insurance company. Others will require a cash down payment if you don't have insurance.

5. Once you've narrowed your choices down, if you have the time and wish to learn more about the emergency rooms in your area, subject each of them to the same scrutiny you used when choosing a hospital:

- Do an on-site inspection. Assess the cleanliness of the premises, the conduct of the emergency personnel, and the waiting time before patients are seen.
- Talk to doctors and people who work at each emergency room, and to patients who have been treated there. Find out their impressions about the quality and nature of care.
- Check on the rating and record of each emergency room. Call or write your local or state health department. The Joint Council for Accreditation of Hospitals includes the emergency room in each of their inspections. You'll be able to learn whether the hospital has ever been cited or punished for health or medical violations in the emergency room.

Once you've considered all of these factors, you'll be able to decide where to go for the treatment of minor emergencies, such as cuts, allergic reactions, stomach pain, and high fevers.

The choice of emergency room for the treatment of major emergencies (at a time when you may be uncomfortable and frightened) involves two additional factors of which you should be aware ahead of time.

1. If hospitalization will be needed after your emergency visit, you may want to go where your doctor is on staff. In this case you'll want to consider the quality of the hospital as well as that of the emergency room.
2. If your problem is severe, such as chest pain or shortness of breath, call the paramedics and let them decide for you. Choosing on your own or attempting to drive there could cost you your life.

Finally, whichever emergency room you choose, or whichever one you're taken to, remember that your rights are identical to those of hospitalized patients. Take the proper steps to ensure them.

1. Read the emergency check-in papers and all consent forms carefully, or if you're too frightened and confused, have a companion read them for you.
2. Realize that you can leave the emergency room at any time you wish.
   Again, the doctor may advise otherwise, but you do have the right to sign out against medical advice ("a.m.a.").
3. Insist on privacy. Your emergency medical situation should never be discussed where other patients can hear or with any other people be-

sides emergency room staff unless you give permission. You should never be examined unless the doors are closed or the curtains drawn.

4. If you're unhappy with any aspect of your emergency care, or you witness the mistreatment of any other patient, call the department of health and report it. Your report might ensure someone else's safety, comfort, and peace of mind and you might help save a life.

TABLE ONE
Circulation and Body Fat Tables

CIRCULATION

Your Blood Pressure

High blood pressure is a "silent killer"—it rarely causes symptoms, until it causes a heart attack or stroke. Pressure varies with age and sex, but "high" is usually defined as greater than 140/90.

Age	"Safe Blood Pressure"
20–30	100/60*–130/80
30–50	130/85–135/85
50 +	135/85**

*Unless it is associated with illness, the lower the pressure, the better.

**Studies have shown that the heart starts to work harder at 135/85, and the risk of disease increases above that point.

Mild elevations respond to diet control more than 50 percent of the time. Because of this and because high blood pressure medications are not without side effects, many doctors will not use medications until the numbers are consistently higher than these—over 145/90 for men over the age of 50; over 150/90 after the age of 70.

Your Pulse

The rate at which the heart beats is affected by many things, but your resting pulse can be a good indicator of your general state of health. Check with the doctor to make sure you're not on medication that could affect your heart rate, then feel for your pulse by pressing two fingers on your wrist.

Beats Per Minute	Condition*
Under 60	Excellent
60–70	Healthy
70–80	Average
Above 80	Unfit; if consistently above 80, check with your doctor.

*Note that a resting pulse under 60 may be indicative of a problem if it represents a change or is associated with symptoms such as weakness, light-headedness, chest pain, or shortness of breath.

Athletes' pulses may be under 50, but any drop to that range in a person who usually has a much higher pulse should be evaluated by the doctor.

All pulses, especially those under fifty, should be checked for regularity. If the pulse is irregular, or is associated with any of the above symptoms, see the doctor as soon as possible.

PERCENT BODY FAT

Although weight tables may help you to decide whether your weight is in the right ballpark, they don't reflect risk due to weight as accurately as "percent body fat."

This number can be calculated by using the "skin calipers," "electrode impedence," or "water immersion" tests, all of which should be performed by an expert.

Increase of Health Risks with Increase in Fat as Percentage of Body Weight

	Men	Risk Increase	Women	Risk Increase
Low	Below 10%	0	Below 15%	0
Ideal*	10%–15%	0	15%–20%	0
Average*	13%–17%	0%–150%**	20%–24%	0%–150%**
Overweight	17%–24%	300%	25%–30%	300%
Obese	25%	500%	30%	500%

*Athletes' "ideals" or "averages" may be significantly lower than the numbers listed, although there is definitely a danger associated with having *too* low a percentage of body fat.

**Since the "average" American is 5 to 10 pounds overweight, the risk may be higher than normal on the upper end of these "average" body fat percentages.

TABLE TWO
Combinations to Avoid

THE EFFECTS OF TOBACCO ON MEDICATIONS

The effect of tobacco smoking on different medicines is believed to come mostly from the effect that hydrocarbons in the smoke have on the liver, where many drugs are metabolized.

Acetominophen   Higher dose may be necessary in smokers.

Antidepressants, tricyclic   Smokers may need higher doses.

Barbiturates (for epilepsy)   Smokers may need higher doses.

Birth control pills   Smokers have an even higher risk of stroke if they take birth control pills.

Blood Thinners (Coumadin, Warfarin)   Controversial effects when mixed, monitor closely.

Doriden   Lower dose is needed.

Inderal and some other heart drugs   Have less therapeutic effect in smokers; higher dose may be needed.

Insulin   Controversial but no proven change.

Talwin (Pentazocine)   Speeds up metabolism; higher doses needed.

Theophylline (asthma medication)   Smokers may need more.

Valium and similar drugs   Higher doses may be necessary in smokers.

Vitamin B$_{12}$ Smoking lowers B$_{12}$ levels; smokers may need more of this vitamin.

Vitamin C   Smokers may need more.

MEDICATIONS DURING PREGNANCY

Medications taken during pregnancy can affect the growing baby directly, by passing through the placenta, or indirectly, through an effect on the mother. The first three months are always the most dangerous, since drugs can affect the development of bodily organs. During the second three months, medications can slow growth and affect the central nervous system.

The last three months are safer, but certain drugs may still affect the baby's breathing, cause early labor, or interfere with normal delivery.

Possible Adverse Effects of Drugs on Fetus When Taken By Mother in First Three Months of Pregnancy

Amphetamines   Affect heart, blood pressure, and nervous system.

Anticonvulsants (used for seizure control)
  Phenytoin   Growth retardation, facial and hand abnormalities
  Trimethadione   Mental retardation
  Valproic Acid   Nervous system defects

Antithyroid medicines (given for overactive thyroid in the mother)   May cause goiter.

Chemotherapies (treatment for cancers)   May cause miscarriage.

Cocaine   May cause miscarriage.

Cough medicines which contain iodine   May cause fetal goiter and thyroid enlargement.

Female hormones (estrogen, progesterone)   Limb and heart abnormalities.

Male hormones (certain steroids)   Masculinization of the female baby.

Phenylpropanolamine (found in diet pills and certain cold medications)   Defects of eye, ear, and penis.

Thalidomide   One out of five get phocomelia, a congenital malformation where upper parts of the extremities are underdeveloped or absent (hands and feet are attached to trunk).

Valium and some other tranquilizers   Cleft palates have been reported.

Vitamin A in excessive doses May cause abnormalities of the urinary tract of the baby.

Vitamin D in excessive doses May cause heart problems.

During the Fourth to Ninth Months

Acetominophen May cause kidney problems for the baby.

Amphetamines Poor feeding, irritability, failure to thrive.

Antibiotics
    Aminoglycosides (Kanamycin) Kidney and hearing problems.
    Chloramphenicol Baby's skin may appear gray.
    Sulfa drugs Anemia, jaundice are possible.
    Tetracycline Yellow teeth, slow growth.

Anticonvulsants Certain medications in this group may cause intrauterine growth problems, bleeding problems, or even addiction and withdrawal in the baby when taken during the second and third trimester of pregnancy.

Aspirin May cause bleeding, especially if baby born prematurely.

Barbiturates Addiction and withdrawal; breathing problems.

Caffeine in excess May cause jitteriness in baby, premature delivery, or low birth weight.

Cimeditine May cause liver problems for the baby.

Cocaine Cocaine addiction and withdrawal in the baby after delivery.

Ibuprofen (Nuprin, Motrin, Advil) May prolong pregnancy and labor.

Isotretinoin Stillbirth, miscarriage, mental retardation possible.

Marijuana and alcohol Lethargy, nervous system changes are possible.

Narcotics Addiction and withdrawal after delivery are possible.

Phenylpropanolamine Decreased oxygen to the fetus is possible.

THE EFFECT OF ORAL CONTRACEPTIVES

Birth control pills (BCP's) can affect and be affected by other medicines. If you take them, you should be aware of the possible interactions.

Ampicillin and Tetracycline   May make breakthrough bleeding more likely when used with BCP.

Dilantin, used for epilepsy and heart disease   May make breakthrough bleeding more likely when used with BCP.

Rifampin, antibiotic used for the treatment of TB   May make BCP less effective.

Tegretol, antiepileptic drug   May make breakthrough bleeding more likely when used with BCP.

THE EFFECTS OF ALCOHOL

In addition to the general depressant effect that alcohol has on the central nervous system, it can also alter the metabolism of drugs by the liver, and their removal from the body by the kidney.

Aspirin   Increased stomach irritation and risk of bleeding.

Blood thinners   Alcohol may be dangerous when used with these medicines (which prolong clotting time), since it can increase the chances of bleeding by its effect on the liver and its capacity to irritate the stomach lining.

Oral diabetic medications   Alcohol enhances the effect; may drop blood sugar too low.

Tranquilizers, narcotics and painkillers   Alcohol may enhance their effect, so the combination is dangerous and potentially fatal. A non-lethal valium dose can rapidly turn fatal when taken with alcohol.

Antiparasitic drugs and certain antibiotics   When used with alcohol may cause nausea and violent vomiting. In addition, alcohol may interfere with effectiveness.

BLOOD THINNERS

These medicines work by interfering with the body's natural blood clotting medicines. They are used for patients with synthetic heart valves, people with "thrombophlebitis," and for certain other patients with heart disease. They can be dangerous if their dose is too high or if they're given to someone who has a bleeding disorder.

Combining them with the wrong medicines without keeping a close eye on the clotting mechanisms can lead to disastrous complications.

Aspirin, Bactrim, Flaglyl (an antiparasitic medicine), Septra (used for urinary tract infections), Tagamet   May all increase the anticlotting effect of blood thinners and cause hemorrhage. Dosage must be reduced if taking any of these while on blood thinners.

Barbiturates and Tegretol   Interfere with medication's action; need higher dose of blood thinners.

OTHER COMBINATIONS TO WATCH OUT FOR

Digitalis (heart medicine) and diuretics   Danger: potassium decrease from diuretics can endanger the heart; take potassium supplements whenever on these combinations.

Digoxin and antacids   More Digoxin may be needed.

Drugs that increase the dangers of a sunburn   Tetracycline, Bactrim, Septra, some birth control pills, diuretics, and Elavil (an antidepressant medicine).

MAO (monoamine oxidane) inhibitors (Eutron, Nardil, and Parnate—used for treatment of depression and certain psychiatric disorders)   Can result in severe, life-threatening high blood pressure when taken with any of the following: Amphetamines, diet pills, Sudafed, many cold and allergy remedies, cheese or wine, liver, pickled herring, salami, sausage, pepperoni, yoghurt, sour cream, bananas, avocados, soybean products, beer, or sherry.

Tegretol and Darvon   Need less Tegretol; it stays in body longer.

Thyroid Hormones   May lose some of their effect when taken with soybeans, rutabaga, brussels sprouts, turnips, cabbage, and kale.

TABLE THREE

If You Need
More Information

You should never hesitate to seek extra help to promote your health and protect your pocketbook.

Whether it's a second opinion about surgery you've been told you need, or simply to clarify something you read in the newspaper, saw on TV or heard on the radio, you need *sources*—people to call and places to write in order to get more information.

The following is a brief list of the resources that I, my patients, and my viewers have found helpful over the years.

PHONE NUMBERS

AIDS National Hotline
1-800-342-AIDS

Alzheimers Disease and Related Disorders
1-800-621-0379
In Illinois: 1-800-572-6037

Cancer Hotline
1-800-4-CANCER

FDA Drug Hotline
1-800-336-4797

Medicare Hotline
1-800-368-5779

National Clearing House for Alcohol and Drug Information
1-301-468-2600

National Second Surgical Opinion Hotline
1-800-638-6833
In Maryland: 1-800-492-6603
Helps locate specialist in your area

Office of Disease Prevention and
Health Promotion
1-800-336-4797
In Washington, D.C.: 202-429-9091
Good referral source on most health
questions

U.S. Dept. of Health and Human
Services
1-800-638-6833
In Maryland: 800-492-6603

U.S. Govt. Printing Office
Washington, DC 20402
1-202-783-3238

U.S. Pharmacopia
1-800-638-6725
In Maryland: 301-881-0256, collect

PAMPHLETS

*A Patient's Guide to Medical Tests Used in
the Diagnosis of Seizure Disorders*
Epilepsy Foundation of America
4351 Garden City Drive
Landover, MD 20785

A Patient's Guide to Nuclear Medicine
Society of Nuclear Medicine
475 Park Ave. South
New York, NY 10016

Alcohol and the Liver
American Liver Foundation
998 Pompton Ave.
Cedar Grove, NJ 07009

Chlamydial Infections
American College of Obstetricians
and Gynecologists (ACOG)
600 Maryland Ave., S.W.
Washington, DC 20024

Diabetes Dictionary
Diabetes Information Clearinghouse
Box NDIC
Bethesda, MD 20205

Growing Children
Human Growth Foundation
4720 Montgomery Land
Bethesda, MD 20814

Health Advisory Program
1909 K St., N.W.
Washington, DC 20049

Health Information for International Travel
U.S. Govt. Printing Office
Washington, DC 20402
1-202-783-3238

High Risk Pregnancy
American College of Obstetricians
and Gynecologists
600 Maryland Ave., S.W.
Washington, DC 20024

Low Back Pain
American Academy of Orthopedic
Surgeons
222 S. Prospect
Park Ridge, IL 60068

Mammography
American College of Radiology
1891 Preston White Drive
Reston, VA 22091

Osteoporosis
American Academy of Orthopedic
Surgeons
P.O. Box 618
Park Ridge, IL 60068

Quackery and the Elderly
Federal Drug Administration
HFE-88
5600 Fishers Lane
Rockville, MD 20857

Seeing Well As You Grow Older
American Academy of Ophthalmology
P.O. Box 7424
San Francisco, CA 94120

Talk About Prescriptions
NCPIE
666 11th St., N.W., Suite 810
Washington, DC 20001

Using Your Medicines Wisely: A Guide for the Elderly
American Association of Retired Persons
3200 East Carson
Lakewood, CA 90714

When You Need an Operation
American College of Surgeons (ACS)
55 East Erie, Chicago, IL 60611

A series of 13 pamphlets on different operations.

ADDRESSES

American Academy of Facial, Plastic, and Reconstructive Surgery
1101 Vermont Ave., N.W.
Washington, DC 20005

American Academy of Family Physicians
1740 W. 92nd St.
Kansas City, MO 64114

American Academy of Ophthalmology
P.O. Box 7424
San Francisco, CA 94120

American Academy of Orthopedic Surgeons
222 S. Prospect
Park Ridge, IL 60068

American Academy of Pediatrics
141 Northwest Point Blvd.
P.O. Box 927
Elk Grove, IL 60009

American Board of Internal Medicine
3624 Market St.
Philadelphia, PA 19104

American College of Obstetricians and Gynecologists (ACOG)
600 Maryland Ave., S.W.
Washington, DC 20024

American Cancer Society
4 W. 35th St.
New York, NY 10001

American College of Radiology
1891 Preston White Drive
Reston, VA 22091

American College of Surgeons
55 East Erie
Chicago, IL 60611

American Diabetes Association
P.O. Box 25757
Alexandria, VA 22314

American Heart Association
535 North Dearborn
Chicago, IL 60610

American Medical Association
535 North Dearborn
Chicago, IL 60610

Arthritis Foundation
1314 Spring St., N.W.
Atlanta, GA 30309

Centers for Disease Control
1600 Clifton, N.E.
Atlanta, GA 30329

Consumers for Medical Quality
P.O. Box 1052
Merced, CA 95341

Food and Drug Administration
HFE-88
5600 Fishers Lane
Rockville, MD 20857

National Clearing House for Alcohol
and Drug Information
P.O. Box 2345
Rockville, MD 20852

The National Hospice Organization
1901 Fort Meyer Dr., Suite 307
Arlington, VA 22209

National Institutes of Health
9000 Rockville Pike
Bethesda, MD 20892

Poison Control Center
2025 I St, N.W., Suite 105
Washington, DC 20006

U.S. Pharmacopia
Problem Reporting Program
12601 Twinbrook Pkwy.
Rockville, MD 20852

BOOKS AND OTHER HELPFUL PUBLICATIONS

American Medical Association, *The American Medical Association's Family Health Guide*. New York: Random House, 1987.

Holleb, Arthur I., M.D., Genell J. Subak-Sharpe, William H. White, Phillip Kasofsky, M.D., eds, *The American Cancer Society Cancer Book*. New York: Doubleday, 1986.

Pinckney, Cathey and Edward R., *The Patient's Guide to Medical Tests*. New York: Facts on File, 1982.

Tapley, Donald F., M.D., Robert J. Weiss, M.D., Thomas Q. Morris, M.D., eds, *Columbia University College of Physicians and Surgeons Complete Home Medical Guide*. New York: Crown, 1985.

MEDICAL TIMES
80 Shore Road
Port Washington, New York 11050
Publishes a list of sources such as these every month

TABLE FOUR

Your Lifetime's Worth of Health Exams

1. This table is a compilation of guidelines suggested by the American Medical Association, American Hospital Association, American Cancer Society, American Academy of Pediatrics. In cases where guidelines are different for the various organizations, the most stringent guidelines are given.

2. Guidelines are for healthy people. Examinations and tests may be necessary earlier and/or more frequently if your personal or family history so dictates.

	Newborn to 5	6–11	12–17	18–24	25–29	30–34
Doctor's History and Physical Examination	Months: 1, 2, 4, 6, 9, 12, 15, 18, 24 Years: 3, 4, 5	6,8,10	12,14,16	Once	Once	Once
Weight	With doctor's examination	With doctor's examination	With doctor's examination	With doctor's examination	Once	With doctor's exam

	Newborn to 5	6-11	12-17	18-24	25-29	30-34
Height	With doctor's examination	With doctor's examination	With doctor's examination	With doctor's examination	Once	With doctor's exam
Blood Pressure	Once after age 3	With doctor's examination	With doctor's examination	With doctor's examination	Every 2½ years to ages 25 to 39	Every 2½ yrs.
Vision	Age 3 and Age 5	With doctor's examination	With doctor's examination	Only if symptoms	Only if symptoms till age 40	Once
Hearing	Once after age 4 unless learning problems	With doctor's examination	With doctor's examination	Only if symptoms	Only if symptoms till age 40	Once
Chest X-ray	Only if symptoms	Only if symptoms	Only if symptoms	Only if symptoms	Only if symptoms	Only if symptoms
Electrocardiogram	Only if symptoms	Only if symptoms	Only if symptoms	Baseline at age 20		Only if symptoms
Blood Sugar	Only if symptoms	Only if symptoms	Only if symptoms	Once	Once	Once

	Newborn to 5	6-11	12-17	18-24	25-29	30-34
Hematocrit (Red Blood Count)	Once in 1st year then at age 4	Once	Once	Once	Once	Once
Blood Lipids: Cholesterol Level, HDL, LAL, Triglycerides	Only if indicated by history	Only if indicated		Every 5 yrs. age 20–60		
Urine Analysis	Once in first year then at age 4	Once	Once	Once	Once	Once
VDRL Test Syphilis	No	No	No	Once sometime after 18 if symptoms		
Testicular Exam	At birth and on entry to school	Only if symptoms	Only if symptoms	Self once/month, age 18 to 50		
Doctor's Rectal Exam	At Birth	None again until age 40				
Proctoscope	None until age 50 unless indicated by history or symptoms					
Stool for Blood	None until age 50 unless indicated by history or symptoms					

	Newborn to 5	6–11	12–17	18–24	25–29	30–34
"Cancer Checkup"	No	No	No	Every 3 years age 20–40		
Rubella Titer (Women)	No	No	No	Once before pregnancy. Best done at age 18		
Tuberculosis Test	Depends on exposure. If high risk, may be necessary as often as every other year.					
Pap Smear	No	No	Every 2–3 years if sexually active	An annual exam until you've had three consecutive normal exams. Then, depending on your symptoms or history, as your doctor advises.		
Pelvic Exam	No	No	Every 2–3 years only if symptoms or sexually active	An annual exam until you've had three consecutive normal exams. Then, depending on your symptoms or history, as your doctor advises.		
Self Breast Exam	No	No	No	Once a month from then		Once a month
Mammography (Or Equivalent)	No	No	No	Only if symptoms or family history		

	Newborn to 5	6-11	12-17	18-24	25-29	30-34
Doctor's Breast Examination	No	No	No	Every 3 years age 18 to 40		Every 3 years to age 40, then every year thereafter

	35–39	40–44	45–49	50–54	55–59	60–74	Over 75
Doctor's History and Physical Examination	Once	Once	Once	Once	Once	Every 2 yrs.	Every year
Weight	With doctor's examination	With doctor's examination	With doctor's examination	With doctor's examination	With doctor's examination	With doctor's examination	With doctor's examination
Height	With doctor's examination	With doctor's examination	With doctor's examination	With doctor's examination	With doctor's examination	With doctor's examination	With doctor's examination
Blood Pressure	At least once a year						
Vision	Once	Once	Once	Once	Once	Every 2 yrs.	Every year
Hearing	Once	Once	Once	Once	Once	Every 2 yrs.	Every year
Chest X-ray	Only if symptoms	Baseline at age 40	Only if symptoms	Only if symptoms	Only if symptoms	Repeat at age 60, then depends on history and symptoms	

	35–39	40–44	45–49	50–54	55–59	60–74	Over 75
Electrocardiogram	Only if symptoms	Repeat EKG age 40	Only if symptoms	Only if symptoms	Only if symptoms		Repeat EKG age 60
Blood Sugar	Once	Once	Once	Once	Once	Every 2 yrs.	Every year
Hematocrit (Red Blood Count)	Once	Once	Once	Once	Once	Every 2 yrs.	Depends on history and symptoms
Blood Lipids: Cholesterol Level, HDL, LAL, Triglycerides	Once	Once	Once	Once	Once	Once	Depends on history and symptoms
Urine Analysis	Once	Once	Once	Once	Once	Every 2 yrs.	Every year
VDRL Test Syphilis	Once after age 18						
Testicles (Men)	Once a month 18–50, then optional. Depends on history and symptoms.						
Doctor's Rectal Exam		After 40, once a year					

	35–39	40–44	45–49	50–54	55–59	60–74	Over 75
Proctoscope				After age 50: 2 normal exams one year apart, then every 3–5 years			
Stool for Blood		Every 2 yrs		Once a year after age 50			
"Cancer Checkup"	Once or twice	After 40, once a yr.		Once a year			
Rubella Titer (Women)	Once before pregnancy—If exposure unknown, not necessary after menopause						
Tuberculosis Test	Depends on exposure and history						
Pap Smear			After the age of 18: annual exam until 3 consecutive normal exams, then depends on history and symptoms				
Pelvic Exam			After the age of 18: annual exam until 3 consecutive normal exams, then depends on history and symptoms				
Self Breast Exam (1 Month)	Once a month	Once a month	Once a month	Once a month	Once a month	Once a month	Once a month
Mammography (Or Equivalent)		First one at age 35–40, every year thereafter					
Doctor's Breast Examination	Every 3 years to age 40, then every year thereafter						

Index